SMARTROLLER® GUIDE
to Optimal Movement

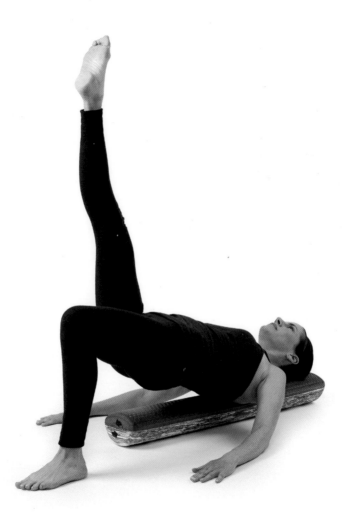

"At the end of the day, a good teacher leaves you
in admiration of yourself, not in admiration of them."

– M. Feldenkrais

SMARTROLLER® GUIDE
TO OPTIMAL MOVEMENT by Stacy Barrows

©2011 by Stacy Barrows

Published by:

OPTP
Tools for fitness. Knowledge for health.
3800 Annapolis Lane, Suite 165
Minneapolis, MN 55447
800.367.7393
www.optp.com

ISBN - 978-0-9843724-5-4

Printed in the United States of America

Every effort has been made to ensure that the information contained in this publication is accurate and current at the time of printing. The ideas, exercises, and suggestions are not intended as a substitute for consulting with your healthcare provider. All matters regarding your health require medical supervision. The manufacturer, author, publisher, or the distributor shall not be liable or responsible for any loss, injury, or damage allegedly arising from any information or suggestion in this publication.

Consult your physician or healthcare professional before starting any type of exercise program, especially if you have health concerns.

contents

THE PROGRAM: The three parts
I. SMARTROLLER BASICS: USING YOUR SMARTROLLER

II. DYNAMIC POSTURE: LINKS AND SITS
THE DYNAMIC ROLLER, LINK BY LINK

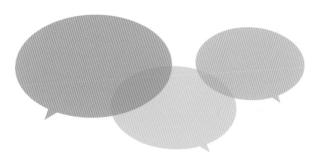

what people say

"The SMARTROLLER offers a new dimension in the use of foam rollers for balance, strengthening and body awareness as part of an overall fitness program. The more rounded side increases the pressure on the spinous processes thereby assisting in the unloading, lengthening and re-alignment of the vertebral bodies and discs in preparation for strengthening of the most important spinal support muscle—the Erector Spinae. The flatter side offers a greater challenge to balance when lying on the roller, thereby stimulating the nervous system and postural support muscles. The SMARTROLLER has added another dimension to my program, the MEEKS Method, in managing the patient with osteoporosis and compression fracture. I use my own SMARTROLLER several times a week in my own personal fitness program."

– Sara Meeks, PT, MS, GCS
Author, International Educator and Clinical Specialist
on Osteoporosis and Intervention

"I also recommend the SMARTROLLER. Here is what I discovered: Every once in a while, an item comes along that promotes the question: 'What did I ever do without it?'. The SMARTROLLER is one of those items. Since I first started working with it, my workouts have been more efficient and more effective. After three surgeries in as many months, this SMARTROLLER has played a major role in my recovery. The exercises given to me by the doctors have become less painful and easier to perform. Not to mention the fact that these same doctors have been amazed by my rapid return to the land of the living.

Before the SMARTROLLER, I was using a standard cylindrical roller to assist in doing stretches and resistance exercises. Balance was always an issue for me but with the SMARTROLLER, although balance plays an important part, I feel more stable and can be more focused on the exercise rather than falling off a roller. I recommend the SMARTROLLER, over any cylindrical roller, to anyone who is serious about achieving their goals and doing their training properly."

– Arthur Rochester, Studio City, CA

"I was looking for a foam roller that I could lie on (facing up) in order to get a good chest stretch. Unfortunately, I have a bulging disk (L4/L5), which makes it painful in the lower back area to lie on a standard 6" foam roller. I sit in front of a computer all day which has given me the beginnings of the rounded shoulder syndrome, so I was advised multiple times to stretch the chest and the front of the shoulders. I've tried the standing doorway and corner stretch, but nothing works as well as lying on top of a foam roller. The good news is that I can lie on top of your SMARTROLLER without any lower back pain in order to complete the stretch. Thank you and best wishes for continued success."

– Roderick Dunham, Ohio

"I thoroughly enjoyed you and your teaching and I learned so much. I use the SMARTROLLER all the time. I developed a "golf" lesson for my husband. The day after his first lesson on the roller he shot his best ever round, improving by 10 strokes! That's when the rest of the guys said, "I want some of that "falling Christ stuff"! Since that lesson I have used the roller with many golfers and they have sung the praises of the SMARTROLLER. Even better, many have their own SMARTROLLER and use it as their warm up to their game. Nothing like a little competition to bring on awareness through movement!"

– Shannon Kennedy
Certified Feldenkrais Practitioner

"I just wanted to take this time to say thank you for inventing the SMARTROLLER! It is the perfect addition to my toolbox! It has such a wide range of applications. It is the smart rehabilitation tool and the smart strength and conditioning tool!"

– Brian Chavarin, MS, ATC, CSCS
Founder & Managing Partner, California Education Connection
www.californiaeducationconnection.com

"I have used a conventional roller; however, the new SMARTROLLER allowed me to adapt, modify and introduce a new realm of possibilities. The SMARTROLLER delivers a much-improved integrated experience of challenge and deeper learning. While, at the same time, the new shape offers many more ergonomic options for the spine, the feet and any gait-related protocol. The roller is bio-mechanically better suited to enhance skill on Pilates equipment. And what I love most is that it leaves no client behind."

– Marie-Jose Blom
Inventor of the Smart Spine,
International and Master Trainer of Pilates

"Foam rollers can be useful supplementary tools for teaching or exploring balance, body awareness and use of self. The SMARTROLLER offers new dimensions of comfort and control, not available from conventional rollers, for experienced as well as beginning roller users. It is a useful addition to any somatic practitioner's toolbox."

– Ralph Strauch, Ph.D.
Certified Feldenkrais® Practitioner
Author of "Low-Stress Computing, Using Awareness to Avoid RSI" and "The Reality Illusion: How You Make the World You Experience"
www.somatic.com

"I have seen many fitness and therapeutic products on the market, and what attracts me most to the SMARTROLLER is how it has such wide application. No other product that I'm aware of allows you to lie on it to improve your spinal mobility as well as stand on it to develop good balance. I see this as having many uses with sports, performance and wellness. I was especially amazed that after doing a body scan and some gentle exercises on the SMARTROLLER, my sacroiliac pain went away."

– Stephen P. Kay, M.D.
Board Certified Orthopedic Surgeon, Beverly Hills, CA

"My passion is finding new ways to make Yoga sessions more accessible to more people. The SMARTROLLER is a useful addition to my Yoga and Feldenkrais® practice. It is a versatile and lightweight tool that gives me many more options for working with my clients."

– Christine Cutbush
Certified Yoga instructor
Certified Feldenkrais® Practitioner
Certified Bones for Life Teacher

"By doing a body scan before and after my use of the SMARTROLLER, I could instantly realize the benefits to my whole body. I felt my core was balanced, and the pain in my back, neck, shoulders, legs and pelvic area had decreased. After using the SMARTROLLER regularly, I feel more flexible, especially when I walk. The pain in my thoracic area has lessened, and I now can sleep on my side without pain.

I consider the SMARTROLLER an essential part of my healthcare. I use the SMARTROLLER in the morning to get me balanced and relieve my pain and energize me for the day. In the evening, I use the SMARTROLLER to relieve my fatigue and pain. I often use it when I have been driving or sitting for long periods.

With the SMARTROLLER, I can take an active role in my therapy in my own home and anytime I want or need to, with good results."

– Sylvia Thatcher, California

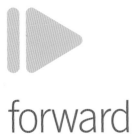

forward

Cognitive science, neuroscience, physiology, medicine, physical rehabilitation and athletic training are a small sampling of many fields in which scientific research into relationships between movement and brain anatomy/physiology are being explored. The information from these studies is being incorporated into many diverse areas including, but not restricted to, treatment plans for patients, training programs for athletes of all levels, movement classes for the public and special education classes.

Recognition of mind-body dynamics is hardly new. Pioneers such as Moshe Feldenkrais, Thomas Hanna, Mabel Todd, Ida Rolf, Bonnie Bainbridge Cohen, Ilse Middendorf and others explored, applied and taught what they learned to colleagues and the general public starting in the middle of the 20th century. Their students and their students' students continue the work today—helping individuals access deeper sensory connections to themselves. Moshe Feldenkrais said that he wished to create ideal learning conditions that would help people develop more flexible minds and intelligent bodies. His approach was to develop heightened awareness through movement by guiding people to tune into sensations of breathing, proprioception and muscular effort that usually exist below conscious levels during normal, day-to-day activities.

What is new are high-tech scientific tools that allow for analysis of structural and functional effects of interactions between the brain and the rest of the body. These include functional magnetic resonance imaging (fMRI), which shows three-dimensional images of brain activity during tasks, and Positron Emission Tomography (PET Scan), which measures the chemical function of the brain among other organs and tissues. Current research supports the benefits of focused attention, balanced muscular tension and improved communication between brain and body.

We also now have more accessible tools like the SMARTROLLER, LINKS and SITS, that may help a wide variety of people enhance awareness of their movement habits, challenge their balance and present them with novel, alternative movements. The SMARTROLLER is a user-friendly foam roller. Its shape provides greater comfort, more flexibility and a safer dismount than traditional cylindrical rollers. The LINKS, used alone or in combination with the SMARTROLLER, widen the range of possibilities even more. The SITS can be used in sitting, standing or lying down.

This book is an essential resource if you have the SMARTROLLER, LINKS or SITS. It is equally valuable to the weekend warrior, elder, texting teen, Feldenkrais Practitioner[CM] and Pilates teacher. The Smart Ideas in this book are presented in a format familiar to those who have studied the Feldenkrais Method® and are easily accessible to those who have not. There is a wide variety of fun, uniquely challenging lessons for people of diverse ages and abilities. I have personally done all of the lessons and each has led me to feel significant changes...as they will for you. Stacy's extensive experience as a physical therapist, Feldenkrais Practitioner, Pilates instructor, personal trainer and lifelong athlete shine through the pages of this book. She emphasizes safety and provides clear, simple, illustrated instructions that are interwoven with at least one way to bring what you learn from each lesson into your daily activities.

I have had the pleasure of working with Stacy as a client and colleague. Her classes and workshops are first rate. She is knowledgeable and passionate about her work. In fact, as a result of our work together, I avoided an unnecessary surgery and, at Stacy's urging, completed a Feldenkrais Professional Training Program. Now I share the benefits of the work with my students, colleagues, family and friends. The SMARTROLLER System is unique. Follow Stacy's guidance and enjoy moving smarter.

– Marci Spiegler, M.S., GCFP,
Adjunct Biology Professor

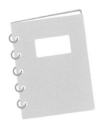

author's notes

I have always been a headlong explorer of movement. My parents love to tell the story of when I was a toddler and jumped into a pool before I knew how to swim. My flailing kept me afloat long enough to be rescued. I can't say that I learned anything from that brief experiment, because several minutes later, my parents watched in horror as I jumped back in. Needless to say, I was quickly signed up for swim lessons. I also grew up riding horses and quickly discovered that, to ride comfortably, you have to match your movement with the motion of the horse. My mother would make me giggle pointing out the actors in movies who were not true equestrians. They were the ones who constantly resisted the horse's motion—the ones who would go home saddle-sore. My dad also contributed to my movement awareness by teaching me how to throw a fastball. His reasoning was that no daughter of his was going to 'throw like a girl'. He helped me realize that there is an efficient way to throw a ball (one that involves the whole body) and an inefficient way (a throw that uses only the arm). Fast-forward a dozen years or so, and I had become a physical therapist. As I see it, the career choice was inevitable, and I have never looked back.

Early in my career, I took the role of body awareness in athletics and my own motor learning for granted. That awareness had helped me become a good swimmer, decent rider and enthusiastic softball player, so I assumed everyone had it. But as a young PT starting to work with patients, I found that many people had problems sensing their own movement and learning from what they felt. This fascinated me and started me on a career-long quest not only to find out why, but also to learn what I could do to change that. Over the years I explored many different neurologically based methodologies to help people learn how to move better. It wasn't until I was introduced to the Feldenkrais Method® that it all made sense. The brilliant engineer and movement scientist Dr. Moshe Feldenkrais had designed a unique experiential educational system that used movement to unlock the powerful learning potential of the human brain.

Experiential learning was not an easy sell for me. Despite my own experiences with movement and movement therapies, I found it difficult to understand experiential learning from a scientific point of view. But slowly, over the course of the four-year Feldenkrais training and countless hours practicing on my own and with patients, it made perfect sense. The Feldenkrais Method helped me refine my own sense of movement and had a powerful effect on my own sense of touch with others. It also prompted my interest in neuroscience and the foundational core of self-learning.

During the Feldenkrais training, I was introduced to foam rollers. In a gadget world, I found that toys helped guide people's attention, so I used them frequently to help people improve their sensory motor awareness and facilitate higher learning. When traditional round foam rollers proved to be too limiting for some people and some types of exercise, I ran headlong into designing and patenting a new foam roller: the SMARTROLLER. After a number of failed attempts to get it made to my specifications, I came in contact with Shari Schroeder and her wonderful team at OPTP. OPTP helped make the dream of a foam roller for *every* body a reality. Today, the SMARTROLLER and related products: SMARTROLLER Links and Sits, are in use in clinics and homes across the country. This book is the companion guide to these Smart products. It attempts not only to show how to use them, but to explain some of the reasoning and inspiration behind them: the principles of physical therapy and the wisdom of the Feldenkrais Method.

I hope you enjoy the process of exploring these movements and thoughts as much as I do.

– Stacy Barrows, PT, GCFP,
PMA Pilates Instructor

smartroller system
A self-guided program of movement re-education

From the earliest stages of life, human beings begin learning how to move. Before our teens, most of our movements are so well-imprinted in our neuromuscular system that they seem intuitive. Without thinking much about it, we can stand up from sitting, navigate a room, throw a ball and so on. Our repertoire of movements and our ability to master new ones expand as we mature. Even before we're fully grown, we are so capable and practiced that, with little thought or effort, we can execute complex patterns, move confidently in unfamiliar settings and quickly recall how to move in ways that we haven't for some time. Most of us only pay close attention to our movement when we need to fine-tune it for some reason—while dancing or putting, for instance, or when trying to avoid pain.

Of course, the human body's wonderful capacity for movement is no guarantee that we will always be able to move with smoothness and comfort. Our neuromuscular system is subject to a host of factors that influence both our ability to move and the quality of that movement. Daily stress, emotional turmoil, accidents and illness take their toll. Overusing or favoring certain muscle groups can produce anatomical imbalances that lead to injury. Sedentary living and aging can also undermine our ability to move well. For any of these reasons, whether we're a teenage texter carrying a heavy backpack, a middle-aged health enthusiast or an active senior, we can develop inhibited movement patterns that compromise our quality of life. We may suddenly find ourselves in pain or unable to do what we once took for granted.

Fortunately, our neuromuscular system is surprisingly resilient and our years of practice with normal, uninhibited movement gives us a firm foundation for improvement. With an effective stimulus and a comprehensive program of guided exercise, you can train yourself to move again with grace and ease. The process is one of gradually becoming smarter about how you move—smart enough to free yourself of bad movement habits, regain lost physical capacity and move comfortably in dynamic new ways. Developing your movement intelligence in this way takes far less effort than you would imagine, and the results can be profound. In a very short time, you can make changes that may last for years.

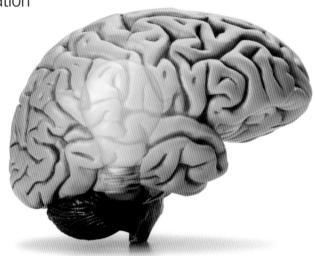

The SMARTROLLER and its companion products, the SMARTROLLER LINKS and SITS, are designed to provide the effective stimulus you need to effect these changes. The SMARTROLLER system teaches you how to use these unique tools with the proper attention to your body while exercising.

The right tool and the proper attention...

While trainers, instructors and therapists frequently recommend foam rollers for stretching or massage, they also have broad applications for movement re-education. To understand their potential and why the SMARTROLLER is particularly useful as a neuromuscular stimulus, think back to your childhood. When we are first learning how to move, the world is a fascinating playground of sensory-motor challenges: stairs, trees, swings, curbs, jungle gyms, balls and skateboards—almost anything big enough to play on or with helps us learn balance and how to adjust our position dynamically in space. As our movements become more refined, we stop needing to challenge our kinetic sensibility with such toys. We spend far more time doing less physically demanding tasks. We sit more and take fewer breaks. Our movement patterns become less varied and more routine. Even if one of those routines is regular exercise, it's likely that we are less active over the course of a day than we were as children.

The SMARTROLLER and its companion products, the LINKS
and SITS are, in a sense, sensory-motor "toys" designed to
reacquaint your body with spontaneous, functional play[1].
They work by stimulating proprioception—the neuromuscular
system's internal feedback mechanism that tells you where you
are in space and the relation of your body parts to the whole.

The SMARTROLLER products stimulate proprioception in ways
that our everyday activities do not. And the effect can be observed
with very little effort in a very short period of time. If all you do
is lie on your back for five minutes with the SMARTROLLER or
multiple SMARTROLLER LINKS positioned lengthwise under your
spine, you will arise feeling less restricted in your chest and back.
If all you do with the SMARTROLLER SITS is to put one under
each sit-bone for a few minutes while driving or at your desk,
you will sit more comfortably, with better balance.

If the initial "aha" experience of using these products is intriguing,
try incorporating them into your daily routine. Just doing these
basic things for a few minutes each day will provide worthwhile
benefits. This is how many people use these products.

While even a few minutes a day pays off, you can accelerate
the kinesthetic learning process and get even greater results
by following the SMARTROLLER program in this book. Over
the course of a few weeks, you'll feel different. Many people
experience a gradual reorganization in their movement
patterns and the way they think about movement. Through
the SMARTROLLER system, you will progressively add more
movement choices to your repertoire. These choices equip you
better to avoid injuries that you could sustain while exercising
or going about daily life. In the long run, as your movement
intelligence increases, you become more able to move with
the comfort, grace and fluidity that nature intended.

Each SMARTROLLER product has unique characteristics that
facilitate the progression of movement awareness and re-education.

[1] Brown, Stuart. PLAY

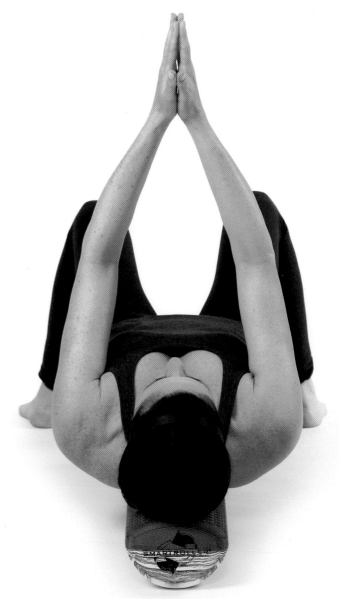

The SMARTROLLER—
the next evolution in foam rollers

For decades, Feldenkrais practitioners and other movement teachers have used cylindrical foam rollers as tools for body positioning and movement re-education. As effective as these tools are when properly used, traditional foam rollers can be too firm for many people to lie on, regardless of age. They can promote over-stretching in certain positions, and the round shape and six-inch height make traditional rollers challenging to mount and dismount. The round cylinder is an unpredictable surface for stand-up balance training and the half-round cylinder commonly used for this purpose may not provide enough challenge when the flat side is against the floor.

The SMARTROLLER is a revolutionary new concept in foam roller design that addresses many of these issues. Made of premium closed cell foam, the SMARTROLLER is comfortable, yet firm and textured for greater grip. It supports your body comfortably whether you lie face down or up, lengthwise or longitudinally, as well as sitting or standing, making it a versatile tool for neuromuscular re-education, with thousands of positional and movement possibilities.

SMARTROLLER's unique shape is the key to its versatility. The dual sides and lower overall height makes it an easy roller to mount and dismount for people of all ages. Because it isn't round like a traditional roller, it doesn't migrate under you or roll away as easily during exercise, either when standing or supine.

The two contours offer different levels of comfort and many options for experimentation. The rounder, more challenging side speeds movement up, while the flatter, less challenging side slows movement down. When the roller is used lengthwise, most people find that the flatter side feels more comfortable along the spine. That's because the less aggressive curve more closely approximates the convex shape of the torso. This gentle shape also eliminates overstretching in the ribs. *And, because it rests closer to the floor, you can lie on it to support the right tension in your body which will allow you to move easier for better discrimination. (Tensegrity concepts; Fuller, Edmondson[2]) Flipped over, with the rounder side up and the flatter side in contact with the floor, the SMARTROLLER has more of an arc providing more stability which creates even more possibilities for movement and balance play.

[2] Edmondson, A. A FULLER EXPLANATION

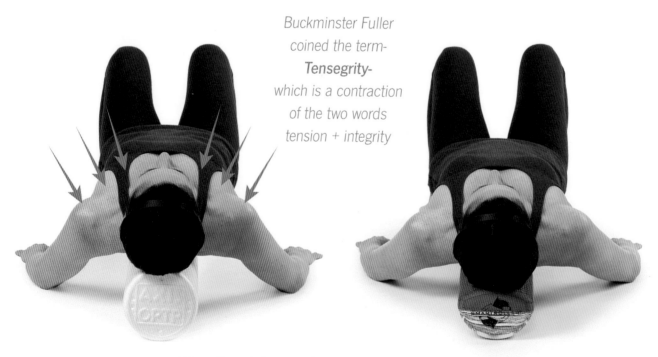

*Buckminster Fuller
coined the term-
Tensegrity-
which is a contraction
of the two words
tension + integrity*

*When there is too much tension in the chest wall, there is
minimal room for the chest and upper body to move on the roller.*

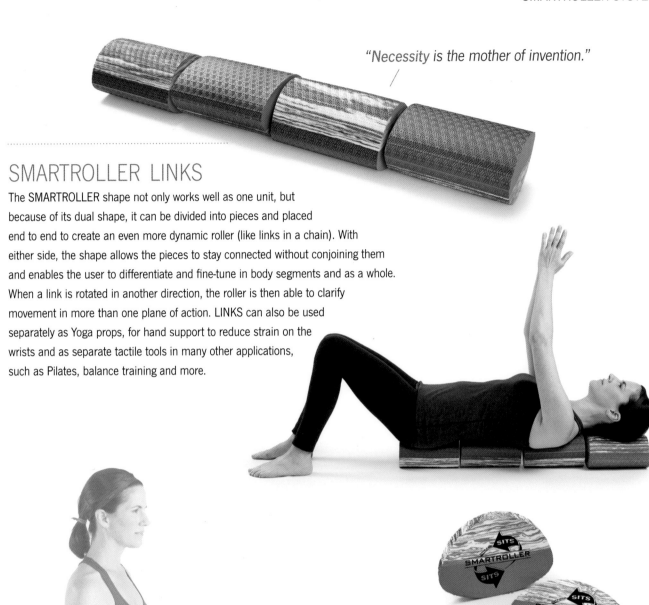

"Necessity is the mother of invention."

SMARTROLLER LINKS

The SMARTROLLER shape not only works well as one unit, but because of its dual shape, it can be divided into pieces and placed end to end to create an even more dynamic roller (like links in a chain). With either side, the shape allows the pieces to stay connected without conjoining them and enables the user to differentiate and fine-tune in body segments and as a whole. When a link is rotated in another direction, the roller is then able to clarify movement in more than one plane of action. LINKS can also be used separately as Yoga props, for hand support to reduce strain on the wrists and as separate tactile tools in many other applications, such as Pilates, balance training and more.

SMARTROLLER SITS

Physical therapists, Pilates and Yoga instructors, and many other movement experts find that balancing your weight on the sits bones promotes an optimal sitting position. The SMARTROLLER SITS – just SITS for short – were designed to assist in this kinesthetic training. The amount of lift along with the shape of the SITS provide easy props to feel for the best solutions to sit in any chair, soft or firm.

Together, the SMARTROLLER products and SMARTROLLER Program help fine-tune your body's proprioception to improve the quality of movement.

the right program...

"Smartroller System" is a step-by-step training program of simple movement sequences, each of which is designed around a functional theme like turning, bending forward or sitting.

The sequences are not exercises as you might think of them, and this is not a workout program in the conventional sense. Exercises in the traditional sense are often thought of as repetitious movements performed while one "tunes out". This training comes from learning through gentle movement cues—"ideas" that can improve the comfort and efficiency of your movement. The program doesn't require athletic skill, aggressive stretching or straining. Since overstretching and pain can be counterproductive to learning, you are never encouraged to push yourself into discomfort. Each idea/sequence is a series of precise, specific movements done at your own pace. The movements are generally small and meant to be done slowly and deliberately.

Movement awareness is an essential part of the program; the goal is to improve your attention to how you are moving. You are not expected to model a particular posture or be shown one correct way to move. You move within your own ability, stimulating proprioception and building kinesthetic awareness by comparing and contrasting different movements in the sequence. By progressively involving more parts of your body over the span of the sequence, you not only improve your range and fluidity of movement, but also develop a better sense of your own capacity and limitations—areas you need to work on because the movement is restricted or rough. As you explore moving in various ways, you will become more skilled at discerning subtle differences in the quality of your movement, and you will add new movement choices to your repertoire.

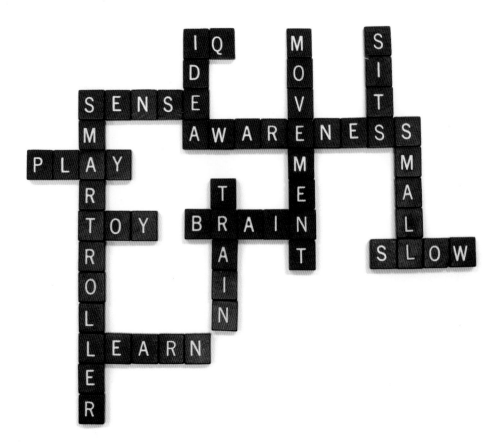

The program itself is divided into three main sections:

1

The first, "SMARTROLLER Basics," is a collection of exercises designed to improve the quality of movement in your whole body. These sequences give you a foundation to help you find optimal strength through better alignment, better organization and reduction in unwanted muscular resistance for a more refined muscular control.

2

The second section, "Dynamic Posture," is a group of exercises to be done with the SMARTROLLER companion products: SMARTROLLER LINKS and SITS. These exercises are directed to less active actions such as sitting and standing which refines posture and creates more dynamic support.

3

The third section, "SMARTROLLER Strength" takes the benefits of learning how to move more efficiently into the realm of fitness. Once you have regained an innate sensitivity to movement, you will be ready for a resistive training workout that can be applied to access a better organization of:

- using large muscle groups in an integrative way for higher performance
- using muscles to work as a coordinated whole

The later sections provide examples and applications that can incorporate better body awareness for better self-care in such everyday actions as lifting, sitting, etc. By making the "SMARTROLLER System of Training" part of your regular physical activity, you will subconsciously start to apply what you've learned in your daily life. You'll use your new repertoire of movement choices to inform the way you sit, stand, walk, drive a golf ball, run a marathon or do a bench press.

Note that while the entire SMARTROLLER program can be accomplished in a just a few weeks, it doesn't have a start and stop. Once you are familiar with the basic concepts, you can pick up at any point, repeat exercises and even customize them to fit your needs. Each time you explore one of the ideas afresh, you bring a new dimension to it—more familiarity, more smoothness, more awareness, sure signs that your movement intelligence is increasing.

This program is not intended to replace any exercise program you are currently using; rather, it is designed to take your workout or training routine to the next level.

On to the program!

"Education never ends Watson. It is a series of lessons with the greatest for the last." – Sherlock Holmes, Sir Arthur Doyle

smart idea program

Before you move on, there are some essentials that will help you capture the best results. The essence of this program is laid out for you to use guided attention with suggested ideas and variations in movement designed to help you learn better. Through this program and through sensory motor learning, you can improve your body awareness, coordination and balance as you refine your movement. "'Sensory motor', because it involves the use of our senses—sight, hearing, balance and touch—in conjunction with movement. 'Learning', because as a result, we learn how to do something new. Sensory motor learning is how all physical learning takes place. It occurs through an information feedback process between your senses, muscles and brain." [1]

First, read through the entire idea, then follow with the movements. Even though pictures are helpful for drawing clues, they can be distracting by diverting your attention to precisely copying the image. Try using the pictures only when you need help in understanding a specific position. Feel confidence in yourself. Remember, this is sensory motor learning, and you are mostly addressing your sense of feel.

This learning process is designed to be completed in steps, so be patient with yourself. Each new idea should take you about fifteen to twenty minutes. Once you are familiar with them, you can benefit from your SMART tools in just a few minutes by simply repeating the parts that interest you. When you repeat the movements on your own, see if you can allow new perceptions to evolve. This will help you recreate the newness of the exercise and direct you to train by using your brain.

[1] Bersin, Reese. Relaxercise.

guidelines for learning

1. Observe your comfort. Pain is not only a signal that tells you that you are doing something harmful; it can also be an attention-getter that distracts you from learning something new. If there is discomfort, try rehearsing the movement mentally or visualizing it. Did you know that you can improve simply by imagining your movements? When you mentally trace the patterns of your movements, you will find that you are able to make even more finely-tuned adjustments.

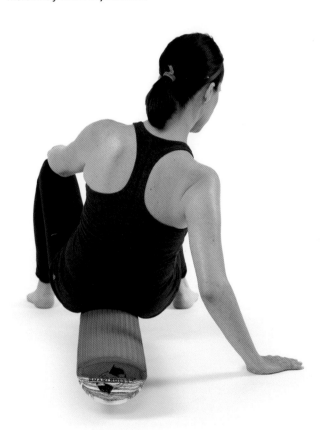

2. Get on the SMARTROLLER. Sit on one end of the roller and lower yourself gently while using one arm to assist you down. Avoid twisting. If rolling onto your back is uncomfortable, or if there is any reason to modify, lie on your side and place the roller up against you to slide up onto it.

3. Scanning: This practice is what helps create the physiological changes in your nervous system that supports new learning. Scanning is done before and after the movement sequences, but can also be done at anytime. By creating this observational process, you will find this practice allows more attentiveness with your movement. Scanning also helps clarify the details of your internal body map. "Formed early in life, they mature with experience and then continue to change, albeit less rapidly, for the rest of your life."[2]

As you read this print, notice how you are sitting. Do your feet touch the floor? Can you notice how your weight is under your pelvis or your buttocks? Is your head tilted to one side, or is it in the middle? Are your shoulders level, or is one higher than the other? How is your breathing? Can you notice these areas without fidgeting?

As you proceed through the book, you will have a more detailed body scan for lying down. Eliminating gravity facilitates more fine tuning to the details of your body position.

4. Small movements, less is more: When you reduce the intensity of your movements, you are able to calibrate and refine how you move. This helps free you from poor movement patterns or habits.

5. Observe your breathing. A resilient respiratory system is adaptable. You breathe differently with different actions. Notice how it feels to breathe when you lie on your stomach, when you run or when you have had a full meal. Your breathing habits may also contribute to more effort, moving against resistance. By attending to your breath in this way, you will be able to observe any unnecessary effort.

[2] Blakeslee, S. THE BODY HAS A MIND OF ITS OWN

"Feldenkrais knew, as did Sherrington, the great neurologist, that most of the brain's activity is inhibitory: it stops, retards or modifies the actions of our more flowing primitive animal brain."[2] – Dr. Norman Doidge author of THE BRAIN THAT CHANGES ITSELF

guidelines for learning

6. Choose variation over repetition to promote learning. While performing these ideas and slightly varying the parts of the movements, you can differentiate and choose which movement choices are better for you. Through variation, you create novel conditions to awaken your brain to help you learn to move in more than one way. (Think of this as your own internal GPS that helps you find alternate and better directions to move.) In the earlier movement sequences, you will be instructed to repeat the movements without a given set of repetitions. This will help you practice exploring the movement. When you reach the exercises for strengthening, the repetitions can be counted, but try not to lose the essence of exploration.

7. Slow down to allow your brain time to register something new and different: Pause between each new movement change to create an opportunity to clarify one movement from the other. How slow? "This question can be answered by another question: how slow do you need to go to discover something new?"[1]

8. Reduce effort and simplify your movements: Excess effort interferes with how you can sense different qualities of movement. Our brains work more efficiently when they are working less, inhibiting unnecessary work. For example, when a person reduces their voice to a whisper, the listener needs to be more attentive to tune out other noises in order to listen better.

9. Avoid stretching: This program is designed to set up conditions for learning. When you go to your extreme range of your movement, you may encounter a pattern that is counterproductive or antagonistic to effortless action. When possible, try these movement ideas without stretching.

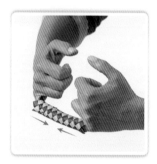 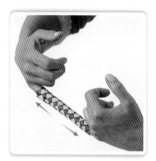

This puzzle provides a way to look at the forces when you pull a complex pattern apart; when you pull muscles in an antagonistic pattern, the results may offer compression or the opposite of release (another tensegrity concept).

10. Reversibility: To reverse a movement is a sure way to improve efficiency. Simply put, it means there is such precision in the movement that you are able to stop a movement at any time and turn the movement around. This can only be done when movement is finely tuned. This also helps you map where you are to allow improvement through pattern recognition.

[1] Yu, Edward. THE ART OF SLOWING DOWN
[2] Doidge, N. ©Norman Doidge
http://www.feldenkraiscentre.com/pdfs/Doidge%20article.pdf

guidelines for learning

11. Concentration vs. Mindfulness: These two states are not the same. Concentrating on the movement outcome can cause unnecessary tension in your body, whereas being mindful, or "bodyful" as Dr. Jon Kabat Zinn calls it, means to direct your attention to the present moment or action. For example, watch how children single-task when they play. You can address this form of learning through a playful attitude and curiosity with movement.[3] Make learning fun and interesting. Practice with a beginner's mind.

12. Take many rests: This provides time to notice the effect of the movement. Our brains need down time to process new information. Think of loading files onto your computer and how you need to pause for the downloading process to take place.

13. To get off the SMARTROLLER: Slide gently to the floor, maintaining contact with the roller as if the roller was a spatula. Then move the roller out from underneath you.

14. Finally, use the roller, LINKS or SITS daily to have the greatest results. Look for subtle changes in your movement to make the effects last even longer. Remember, it is not the movements themselves that make the improvements; what you learn from them makes the changes. There is no limit to improvement.

NOTE: As with any exercise system or device, always clear the use of the SMARTROLLER products with your health provider. Never do movements into pain; there is no place for the "no pain, no gain" approach. Instead, follow the "no pain, more gain" approach to support better learning.

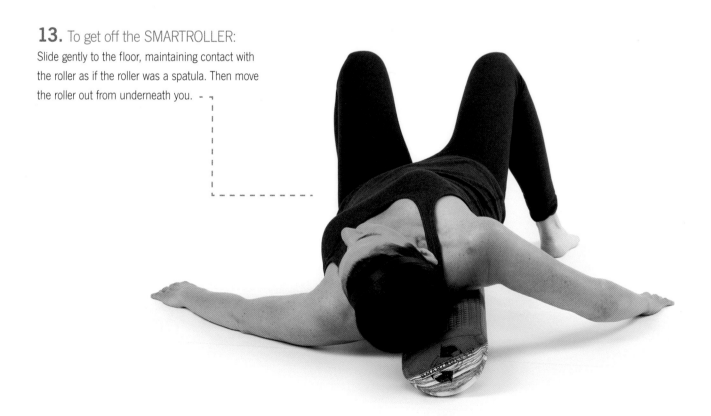

[3] 5 Brown, S. PLAY

"...In essence, creating neural networks, and indeed the process of neuroplasticity, requires focused attention." – David Perlmutter, MD, FACN, ABIHM

body scan

This body scan should be used before, during and after the movement "ideas" to assess any changes and to help you establish a better sensitivity to your body alignment and sense of movement. This is what sets this approach apart from other ways of training. By noticing yourself in these details, you will learn to fine-tune your movement, posture and alignment.

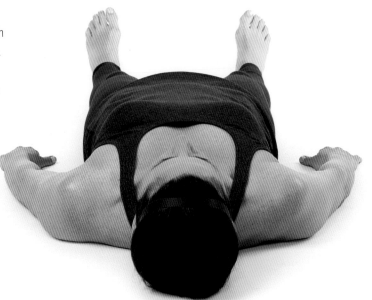

Lie on your back and allow your legs to lengthen on the floor and your arms to rest alongside yourself.

- Notice how your two legs are resting. Which leg is longer, heavier and more in contact with the floor?

- Observe where your legs do not make contact and measure the size of that space with your imagination.

- Which way are your toes pointing; does one leg turn out more than the other, and how does this relate to the heavier leg?

Can you answer these questions by "feeling" how you are resting instead of moving or looking at yourself?

Which way are your knees pointing; are they wider than your hips or closer in than your hips?

How is your pelvis resting on the floor; is your right buttock making more contact than your left buttock?

How does the end of your spine rest on the floor; is your tailbone or your sacrum (the flat bone above your tailbone) touching?

What is the space like under your low back; how much space is there and where does the spinal contact begin and end?

How does the rest of your spine make contact with the floor; can you feel the curves your back makes as you move up the spine in your awareness?

Do you feel your ribs making contact, and how do they compare from left or right?

How do your shoulders rest on the floor, and which shoulder is in more contact?

How do your shoulder blades compare in shape with the contact they make with the floor? If you were to lower the ceiling to reach your shoulders, which shoulder would be touched first?

How much space is under your neck; is it larger than your low back or smaller?

Where is your head resting; where is the point of contact with relation to your ears; are you resting closer to one ear than to the other?

How are your arms resting; which is longer; which has more contact; how does the contact with the fingers compare from left to right?

Finally, how does your breath influence your overall contact with the floor? Does the contact change when you inhale? Exhale?

"Make curiosity your goal." – M. Feldenkrais

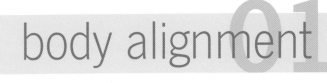

body alignment 01

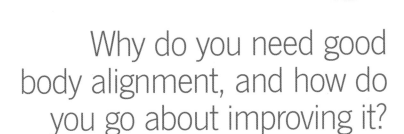

Why do you need good body alignment, and how do you go about improving it?

Ideal alignment allows you to balance more easily in many directions, which helps you sustain dynamic control with your posture. When you move efficiently, your body moves as an integrated network using a self-alignment system. Because this is not a static process, you need to tune this process through movement. Feldenkrais describes efficient movement as "freeing an action of wasted energy".

Optimal alignment also requires a central support integrating your pelvis with your spine. When you use the SMARTROLLER with the action of rocking and focused attention to the effects of gravity, your spine is free to move from left to right to create this central organization. Through this process, you will free unwanted muscular tension and reduce wasted energy.

start with the body scan
Orient the roller solid side up: SU

- Lie on the roller with the support under your head and pelvis. Note the natural curves in your body with the sensation of the roller against your back. Don't try to change the curves, just notice without doing.

- Next, gently tilt your right leg out to the right and back. Do only a small amount of movement to allow you to balance on the roller easily.

- Observe how your body does this movement. Move slowly and smoothly, noticing the details of the movement. Can you sense if your leg moves separately from the rest of your body, or does your body immediately move with the leg? Try it both ways, each time moving more smoothly. How do they compare? Pause.

- Repeat this a few times to observe how your body moves. Note: The return of movement has just as much importance as the actual movement, so stay attentive throughout the sequence. Pause or rest.

- Now start to tilt the left leg to the left and back. Repeat this movement a few times and attend to how you start each movement. Where do you begin the movement?

- Now you have two sides to compare with. Which side is easier? Which side seems more fluent, smooth and continuous? Try different variations. Let your body move slowly with each leg in a synchronous form. First the leg moves, then your pelvis, on up to your opposite shoulder. Move your body in one piece. Which way seems more familiar, natural? Rest on the roller.

- Next, alternate your legs. First the right leg, then the left leg. Be very clear when one leg stands and when one leg moves. The leg that is not moving should be still, not rigid. There is a moment when you switch between movement and stability between your two legs. Are you able feel your spine and how it connects to your pelvis? Pause.

- Return to tipping your legs, alternating right to left. Through this easy rocking motion and adjusting with a simple balance you will help re-align your skeleton.

  Notice what your feet are doing. Allow them to respond to the tipping. First allow them to tip with the legs, then keep them flat on the floor. How does this change the movement? Does your head move? Let your head gently tilt towards the leg that tips out a few times...then the opposite direction a few times. Then leave your head in the middle. How do these movements compare?

- Continue the rocking movement and notice how your eyes participate with the movement. Try to focus your eyes on a spot on the ceiling. Does this slow the movement or diminish it in any way?

- Now allow your eyes to go in the direction that your legs are moving. Has this become any easier? Pause in the middle. Notice if you are more relaxed over the roller. Do you feel that more of your body is draped over the roller? What is your breathing like?

- Before you roll off the roller, see if you can rehearse this mentally. Once you are ready, roll off the roller. Can you slide off the roller while breaking very little contact with it? Repeat the body scan and notice if there are any changes.

Think of how you move an icon on your computer. If you lose contact with the icon, it no longer moves.

- Are you more symmetrical? Is there an empty space where the roller once was? Do you feel more of your body in contact with the floor now? Are you more aware of the midline of your body after using the SMARTROLLER?

- Get up slowly with the same gentleness you did with the roller and notice your standing alignment. Are you taller? More weighted on your feet? Do you feel more balanced?

- Walk around to allow time to assume this new easy upright posture.

- See if you can keep this sense of yourself and are able to imagine where the middle of your body is when you sit, stand or walk around.

This movement is a basic action when we shift our weight with walking. When we walk with a healthy spine, our vestigial tail wags.

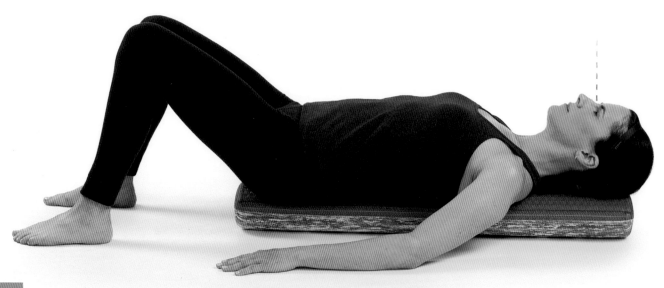

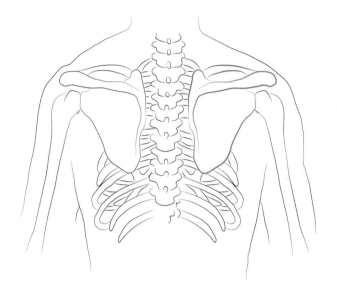

The anatomy of your shoulder is designed to provide a wide range of motion, allowing for a broad range of use of your arms.

However, if done poorly, these mechanics may present challenges while you sit at a desk, lift objects or perform finely coordinated skills with your hands. When the SMARTROLLER is flipped over, the oval shape will support your upper body, allowing your shoulder blades to move easily on your back. This idea will help restore a balanced muscle support in your arms and full body.

start with the body scan
Orient the roller solid side down: SD

- Lie on the roller, solid/flat side down. The roller will now have less rocking motion and a sharper curve in contact with your body. This supports the anatomical curve of your back and allows for a better resting position of your shoulder blades. If this is too uncomfortable, first try a rolled blanket to feel the following movements without any discomfort. (Refer to the basics about learning without pain.)

- Rest on the roller with your knees bent and position your legs where you can balance easily. Lift your arms straight up and bend your elbows to form a rectangle shape with your arms.
- Think of a rectangular box made up of lines drawn between your two shoulder blades, your upper arms and your forearms. Notice which hand is on top. Now switch your hands so the opposite hand is on top. Notice the difference.

Which seems more familiar? This will help illuminate how everyday movement habits become unconscious. We choose them without having to think about them. The familiar way may often be confused with being the best choice; in order to discover the correct choice, variations performed for comparisons are helpful.

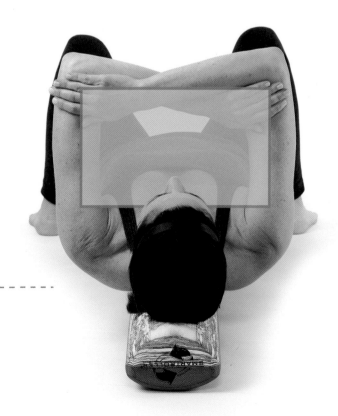

- Return your arms to your original formation. Now keep your arms in this shape and, without deforming the rectangle, lift them towards the sky. Don't extend to your full range of motion—only move enough to avoid stretching. This allows for better sensitivity.

- Return your arms to the rectangle position; change your arms so the opposite arm is on top. Repeat the lifting of the rectangle. Repeat this several times and notice how this compares.

  Is there a difference? Is your head responding to the movement?

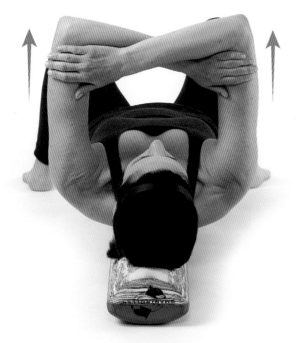 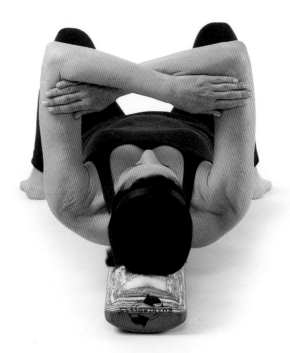

- Repeat this movement several times to notice the differences between your two arms.

  How do they compare? Which arm moves easier? Be sure to allow the movement to travel towards the floor, allowing your shoulder blades to slightly wrap around the roller.

- Lower your arms and rest. How is your breathing at this time? Are there any changes?

NOTE: When movement is performed to the full range, to the point of a stretch, there is a reflex that is stimulated called the stretch reflex. This may seem like it feels good but when the stretch reflex is signaled, it returns to the old habits and overrides any opportunity to try something new.

- Lower your arms to the floor and rest on the roller. Bring your arms back into the original rectangle position. Now tilt the arm rectangle slightly to the right. You will need to rotate the rectangle to the right. Again, can you do this without deforming the shape of the rectangle? (see diagram)

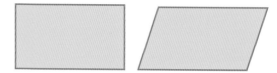

- Keep your balance easy. Return to lifting your arms towards the sky, but with your arms oriented slightly to the right. As you repeat this movement, your shoulder blades will be traveling at different lengths and different speeds. This is similar to running around a racetrack, where one has an inside advantage. Do this several times, then rest with your arms down.

- Return your arms back to the center and now tilt them, in the rectangular position, slightly to the left. Which one is more difficult? Easier? Now repeat lifting the rectangle towards the sky. Move slowly so you can make the movement smoother through each repetition.

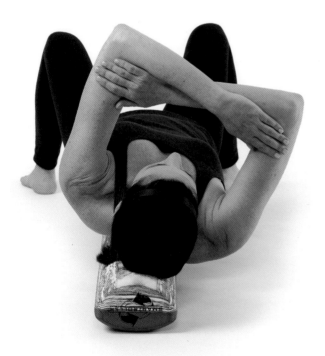

- Rest your arms at your sides. Now gently roll off the roller. Notice how you rest on the floor.

  Can you feel a change in the shape of your upper back?

- Return to the roller and bring your arms into the rectangle position. This time place the opposite arm on top—the less familiar position. Now tilt the rectangle upward, towards your head so your arms are just over your eyes, and lift your arms in this direction to feel how this compares with the previous

movement. Allow your shoulder blades to slide down your back towards your feet. Repeat this several times, making each movement smoother.

How do your two arms move and how do they compare?

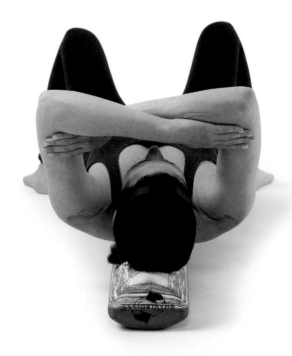

- Rest your arms by your sides. Pause for a minute and then gently slide off the roller.

  Return to the body scan. How is it different? Is there a sense that your upper back is wider? What is your breath like? Is your spine in more contact with the floor?

- Stand up and walk around and allow your arms to dangle freely as you walk. Notice if your walk has changed. Does your upright posture feel taller?

As you are able to sense your shoulder blades better, you will be able to unravel unnecessary neck and shoulder tightness when you are sitting, standing or walking. See if you notice other patterns in your shoulders. Are there other geometric shapes you are able to sense when you hold an object and push or pull something? Like a circle or triangle?

Often when you aim to release tension in your neck, you're really just exercising it. Whatever made your neck stiff will return once the temporary fix goes away. By learning to use more than one movement pattern, you will have more choices to choose from and allow yourself better movements to reduce strain.

Try this: Take a jar and screw off the lid. Do this in as many ways as you can to see what the possibilities are. Now, hold the top of the jar still and rotate the bottom of the jar to unscrew it. Because this pattern is far less familiar to us, we often overlook this possibility.

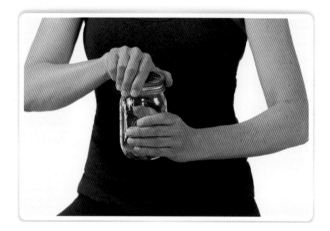

This next idea will help you create new ways to rotate your body on your neck as an alternative to moving your neck on your body.

Lie on your back and start with the Body Scan. Roll your head gently from side to side. Move slowly enough to see which side moves better.

Orient the roller solid side Up: SU

• Lay the roller on the floor and lie on your left side, resting your face on the flat side of the roller. If this is uncomfortable, place a small soft foam pad or pillow on top of the roller. Put your arms on the floor in front of you with your elbows out straight and your palms on top of each other (forming a triangle with your two arms).

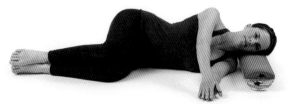

• Without bending your elbow, lift your right arm in the air and point it towards the ceiling. Then, return your right arm back on top of the left arm.

Repeat this several times and notice how you do this and what the weight of your arm feels like. Observe how you breathe. Is your movement smooth? If not, where does it seem to be jerky? Rest your arm back down on top of your left arm.

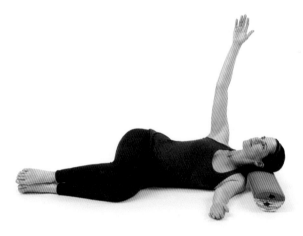

• Now, slide your right hand on the floor away from you, as if you are reaching past your left hand. What stops your movement or resists you from going farther without strain? Do you feel your upper body start to roll in the direction you are reaching? Pause.

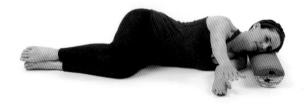

• Repeat the same movement of sliding your hand forward and then start to lift your hand off the floor towards the ceiling. Notice how this moves your shoulder blade. Repeat this several times.

Notice how your eyes respond to this movement. Follow your right hand with your eyes and allow your head to roll passively in the same direction. How does this affect your movement? Rest on your side with your arms down.

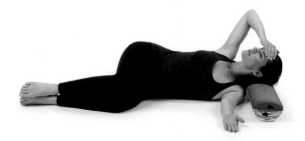

• Place your right hand on your forehead and slowly roll your head to the right, making sure you keep your head and arm moving together. Reduce your movement in half to allow for a smooth guided motion. Notice the relationship to your left arm on the floor.

   As you roll in this way, see if you can sense your left arm getting longer. Can you track both your right arm and your left arm at the same time? Can you sense that you are turning in between your shoulder blades? Think of this turning motion like a bank's revolving door. In order for the door to turn, both sides must be allowed to move and rotate.

• Rest in the middle.

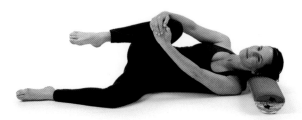

• Take both hands and hold onto your right knee. Gently lift your right knee towards the ceiling. Allow the rest of your body to start to roll a little. Go only so far that the opposite leg can stay on the floor and then position the right leg back on top.

• Repeat this several times. Be sure to breathe throughout the movement. Rest.

• Repeat lifting your right arm in the air towards the ceiling. Is it any easier?

• Slide the roller out and roll onto your back. Roll your head from side to side. How do they compare now? Which side is easier?

• Now lie on your right side and rest your head on the roller, placing your arms out in front as before. Lift your left arm towards the ceiling. Does this side seem different? Repeat this several times but reduce the movement down to half of the range of motion from before. Rest on your side.

• Return to the same movement and focus on something in front of you. As you lift your left arm up in the air, keep your eyes on the same point. Does this affect the movement of your head?

   Can you allow your head to rest comfortably on the roller as you do the movement? Repeat this several times. Again, move to only 50 percent of your available movement. Rest.

• Rest your left hand on your forehead; slowly roll your head to the left, again making sure you move your head and arm together. Observe how this turns your spine in a sequential motion, like a spiral staircase. Come back to the middle and repeat this slowly several times, pausing in the original position.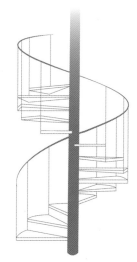

• How are your eyes moving? Can you start the movement with rolling your eyes in the same direction and following with the rest of your body?

• Now, move the roller out of your way and roll onto your back. Gently roll your head from side to side to see if this movement has become any easier.

• Stand up and see if it is easier to look around. Walk outside, making sure to look at the scenery to reinforce any changes you might experience when you look around. Now that you can feel the vital connection of your eyes to the movements of your head and neck, explore looking around with your peripheral vision (the outer edges of your field of vision). You may be able to sense this way of moving with easy turning now that you have less body tension.

See if you can find more solutions to turning your head by moving in alternative ways—e.g., focus on an object in front of you and twist your body without turning your head-compare this with keeping your body still and turning your head. In what other ways can you accomplish this same change of habit?

breathing dynamically

You use many breathing patterns throughout your day. No single pattern is suited for all your activities. Ideally, you need an adaptable respiratory system so your breathing can supply what you need for the moment. Here you will play with a variety of movement patterns while observing how you breathe. The intention is not to find one perfect way to breathe but to create a better sense of flexibility with optimal breathing.

start with the body scan
Orient the roller solid side up: SU

- Lie on the roller, letting it support your head and pelvis. Note the natural curves in your body with the sensation of the roller against your back. Observe how you are breathing. Did you take a large breath in automatically? Try to notice without doing.

- Follow the rhythm of your breath for a couple of minutes. See if you can create the image of a rib basket instead of a stiff rib cage. As you imagine this, create the image of soaking the basket reeds to soften them to allow easy motion.

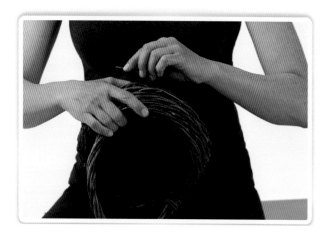

- Balance quietly on the roller and place your hands on your belly. Follow the movement of your breath with your hands. Next, place your right hand on your chest and feel for any movement in your chest. Compare this with your belly movement. Follow this for a few breaths with your hands over your chest and belly.

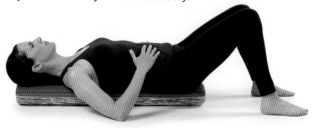

- Next, breathe in and gently draw your belly in, then breathe out normally. Without strain or any exaggeration in your inhalation, repeat this a few times. Observe how your ribs feel in the front and in the back where the roller touches them. Are you more aware of yourself three dimensionally? Think of this space as an elastic beaded bracelet.

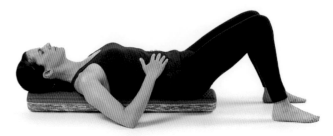

- Return to your regular movement with your breath.

- Next, when you breathe in, expand your belly and repeat this for a few breaths.
  You may notice that one way is easier than the other. Which way seems easier?

- Now, alternate your movements with your breath—one with pulling in your belly when you breathe in, then one with pushing out your abdomen when you breathe in—and do this a few times, noticing how this feels in your ribs, belly and your contact with the roller. Continue to reduce your effort as you do this. Pause and place your hands back on the floor. What does your breathing feel like now?

"Breathing is the simplest thing in the world until you start thinking about and analyzing it." – Eric Franklin

- Return your hands, and this time place your left hand on your chest and your right hand on your belly. Breathe in normally, then breathe out as you push your belly out. Repeat this several times and notice any differences in the way this feels. Is it any easier to coordinate your breath in this way? Return to your familiar breathing pattern. Roll off the roller and rest on the floor. Observe your contact with the floor now.

- Return to the roller and place your left hand on your chest and your right hand on your belly. When you breathe out, pull your belly in. Does this affect your breathing? Does this assist you in any way? Repeat this several times. Notice this with your hands. Return to your regular breathing and rest your hands on the floor.

- Leave your hands on the floor and combine breathing in and pulling your belly in, and breathing out and pushing your belly out. Continue this see-saw breath and repeat this several times, making the transition of breaths smooth and rhythmical.

- Rest. Without interfering with your breathing, slide to the floor. Move the roller out of the way and scan your contact with the floor. Notice any changes? Is there a difference in how you are breathing?

- Turn the roller so the solid side is up; lie on your front side on the roller. With your head slightly off the roller, place a small rolled up towel under your forehead. Observe what this feels like when you breathe. Bend your knees, rest your knees on the floor and repeat the see-saw breath. Be gentle. If for any reason resting on your front side is uncomfortable, slide onto the floor and do this without the roller. Continue the see-saw breath a few times. How does this affect the movement of your back, chest and ribs?

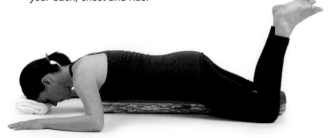

- Now, slide onto the floor and roll onto your back. Notice how your breath is. Does your breath seem any easier?

- Try this in varying positions with the roller-such as sitting, side-lying or placing the roller under your pelvis. Experiment with these positions to see how this affects how you breathe. Observe your breathing patterns throughout the day.

How can you create more opportunities to observe your breathing habits? Observe how you respond with other breathing styles, such as sighing or pushing out bursts of air while sneezing, coughing and laughing.

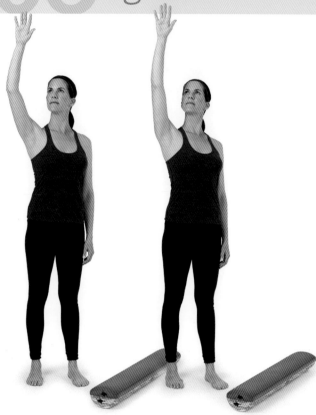

Orient the roller solid side up: SU
Scan your contact with the floor (Body Scan)

- Place the roller on the floor about 5 inches from the wall. Lie on the roller with your knees bent and your feet on the floor. Rest your arms by your sides.
  Observe your breathing and how easily you balance.

- Bend your arms at the elbows so your hands are pointing to the sky, relax your wrists and fingers to direct your palms upward, as if you had to hold a platter on each hand.

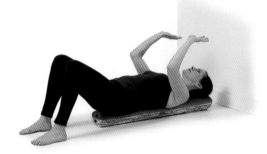

- Now, lift your arms in the air, keeping your elbows bent, and continue this until you are able to touch both hands to the wall behind you. Your fingers will be pointing downward. Your arms should be bent, so adjust your position if you are too far from the wall. Can you pause in this position?

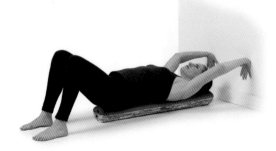

- Press gently with both hands into the wall. Can you allow your spine to follow the movement? Can you allow your chest to be responsive to the movement without becoming rigid?
  How do you perform this movement? Does your back gently arch? Notice how your feet respond to the change in movements. Repeat this a few times. Lower your arms and rest.

Reaching overhead is a complex organization for your whole body. Besides the obvious demands on the shoulder, your legs and torso are critical in supporting your arms for this task.
Think of the tension that would occur at your shoulders when you reach up if you were wearing suspenders or if your shirt were to stay tucked in.

This next sequence will help you find new ways to perform this movement more efficiently. With the use of a wall for pressure and the SMARTROLLER, you will re-create similar strategies to the ones you learned in early childhood development by using your arms for crawling and pushing off.

Before you start with the Body Scan, stand up and reach overhead. Try it with both arms, then with one arm at a time. Observe how easy it is and how your arms compare.

Pushing hands is a two person training which helps teach
tai chi students to neutralize their attackers brute force.

- Return your arms to the wall as before. Expand your abdomen.
  Gently protrude your belly and notice how this allows you to
  arch in the small of your low back.

  *Repeat this several times and synchronize this with pushing
  into the wall. Pause and rest.*

- Now widen your legs so they are farther apart—about 6 inches
  each. Gently press into the wall and see how this affects the
  movement in your spine.

- Lower your arms and roll off the roller to rest on the floor.

- Return to the roller and place just your right hand on the wall.

  *Gently press into the wall with your right hand. How does
  your low back respond to only one arm pressure? Notice
  what your head does. Keep repeating the movement. Track
  the force of movement through your whole body; see if you
  sense pressure changes to your opposite foot. Remember,
  the lighter the pressure (less effort), the more magnified
  your senses are.*

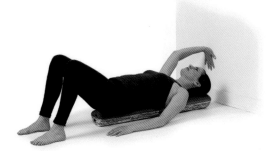

- Next, allow your head to roll with the movement. Do you
  roll to the left, right or not at all? Which direction is easier?
  Now, return to your original direction for comparison.

  *Can you make this movement smoother? Try alternating the
  movement as you make the movement easier. What do your
  eyes do? Pause in the middle. Lower your arm and rest.*

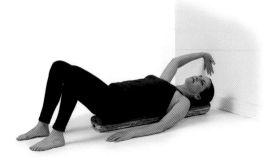

- Try this with your left arm.

  *Do you remember how the right arm felt from before?
  What are the differences between the two sides? Lower your
  arm and rest.*

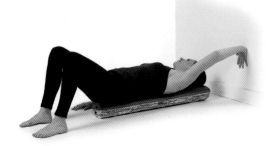

- Bring both arms back to the wall and press with both hands
  as before. Has this changed? The pressure into the wall is
  not to create tension with force, but to permit the force to
  move through you. Similar to the concept of "pushing hands"
  in Tai Chi, you are moving your arms to be responsive to
  the moment.

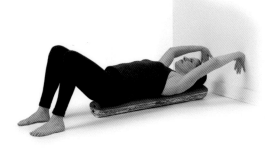

- Now, lift your legs in the air, one at a time, and bend at the
  knees into the table-top position (your hips and knees are at
  90˚). See if you can breathe easily while holding this position.
  Balance yourself by using your hands to support yourself in
  your middle. Think of this as a hand stand and using your
  hands for sensitivity to make fine adjustments.

  *Can you do this without tensing your neck?
  Tightening your jaw?*

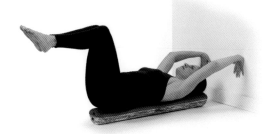

- Keeping your balance, tilt your left leg a little out to the side. Again, allow your arms to assist you.

  How does this affect your balance? Return your leg to the middle and try it with the right leg out to the side, taking note of which side is easier. Lower your legs and arms one at a time to the floor and rest.

- Return your arms to the wall and gently push into the wall as you did in the beginning. Has this movement changed for you?

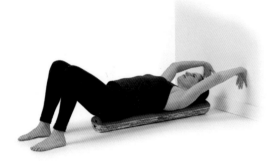

- Now, lift your legs back into the table-top position. Challenge your balance a little by moving your legs one at a time in different positions. Observe how each position varies your balance reaction in your arms and through your whole body. Listen with your hands for fine tuned balance reactions. Think of the sensation you feel when you balance on one foot. You are now having a similar experience to notice changes in your hands.

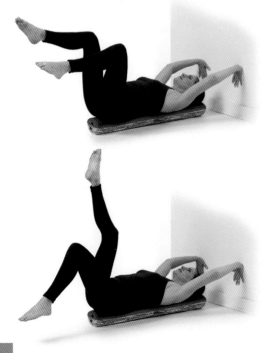

- Lower your arms to the floor; gently slide off the roller and rest on the floor. Notice how your body rests and feels compared with how it did at the beginning.

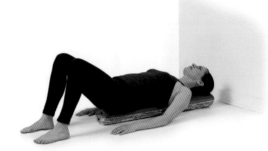

- Stand up and reach overhead with your right arm, then your left arm. How does this compare to before? Lift both hands in the air and see if you are more aware of your feet pushing off of the floor to make this movement happen. Can you see how this allows you to reach overhead without isolating your arms or straining your neck or back?

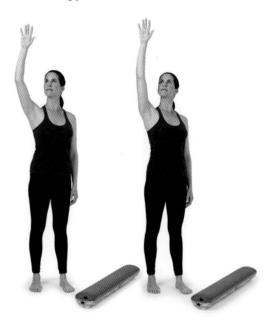

What other activities would benefit with full body lengthening in your daily life? Swimming? Pushing a heavy object in any direction? Reaching towards a high shelf? Now that you've found ways to support your arms with better ground support, see if you can find ways to apply these mechanics with your arms when you perform daily tasks, such as laundry, dishes or driving. Notice that, by distributing the effort more evenly in your body, you lessen the strain in your arms.

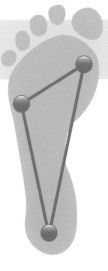

 # balancing while lying 06

Our balance is linked fundamentally to everything we do. We need to practice skills that support and nurture dynamic balance throughout life.

By reducing the challenges of standing balance, you will attend to subtle changes in how you recover your balance, making it easier to make fine-tuned adjustments. The smallest distinctions you notice with your breathing will direct your attention to a very finely tuned balance.

start with the body scan
Orient the roller solid side up or down:
SD (easy) or SU (advanced)

• Lie on the roller, letting it support your head and pelvis. Note the natural curves in your body with the sensation of the roller against your back.

Observe your breathing – just notice without doing. How quiet can you rest on the roller without stiffening? Notice where you place your feet on the floor. Think of each foot having points of pressure, like a tripod: pressure at the knuckle of the big toe, the knuckle of the little toe and the heel. Compare how the contact is under both feet.

• Now slowly tilt your body a small amount on the roller to feel the adjustments under your feet. When you tilt to the right, do you feel how your weight adjusts under your right foot? Your left foot? Then, tilt your weight slightly to the left, noticing the effects under each foot. Pause in the middle.

Feel how your arms are resting on the floor and how they compare.

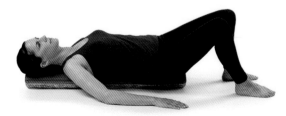

• Return to rocking from side to side, noticing the subtle changes in your arms, shoulders, chest and spine.

Pause in the middle. What helps you find the middle of your body? Can you feel how different parts of you can help direct you to the middle?

• Next, lift your right foot off the floor about one inch to feel how your full body adjusts to the change in position.

What is balancing you at this point? Did you stop breathing? Slowly return your foot to the floor. Where is the first point of contact with your right foot as you touch the floor? Repeat this five to six times to make very clear distinctions between balancing from three areas in your body compared to four areas.

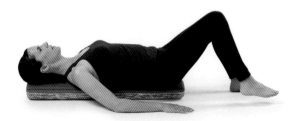

• Try this with your left foot.

How are the two sides different? Is one side easier? Repeat this several times to observe the subtle changes in the pressure under your right foot and then with the placement and return of your left foot. Observe any gaps or pauses in your breathing. Rest, with both feet supporting your balance, and notice if it seems easier.

Recent studies have shown significant improvement in balance using the Feldenkrais Method®.
☞ Go to: http://www.gettinggroundedgracefully.com.au/research.html#balance

- Lift your left leg in the air with your knee bent (your foot is hanging down) and place your right hand on your left knee to support it. Adjust your right standing foot to secure your position. Avoid stretching and hold your knee while keeping your elbows straight.

  Notice how you balance. Does your right foot feel secure? See if you can quiet yourself in this position. Reduce any tension in your face, jaw and chest.

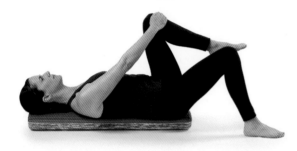

- Keeping your left leg in the air, lift your left hand off the floor, bringing both hands together to hold your left knee.

  Can you balance quietly like this? Where do most of your balance adjustments come from? Do you stiffen anywhere as you are challenged? Gently return your left foot to the floor, lower your arms and notice where you place your foot. Has the placement of your left foot changed? Rest on the roller.

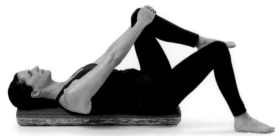

- Lift your right leg in the air and reach for your knee with your left hand, holding your knee in the air. Relax your right knee, allowing for your right foot to hang down.

  Is this side easier or more challenging? Look for the differences regarding how your body adjusts to the change in your legs.

- Now lift your right hand from the floor and hold your right knee with both hands.

  How is your left foot balancing on the floor? Is there an adjustment you can make to balance more easily? Arrange

your left foot to support your balance with less effort. Maintain this position and notice your breathing. Lower your leg and rest.

- Return to your original movement and lift your left leg while you support it with both hands. Has this changed or is it the same way you did it before? Now, look from right to left, slowly enough to notice any adjustments with your balance.

  How do you do this? Do you move your head with the movement? Try it first with only your eyes, then include rolling your head in the same direction as if you wanted to look at something. Follow it from side to side. Is there a difference from right to left? Rest in the middle and lower your left leg to the floor.

- Try this with your right leg; first hold your knee with the opposite hand and then add your right hand. Gently roll your eyes from side to side, and make the movement smoother each time. Allow your head to follow.

  Is it different with this side? Now focus your eyes on the ceiling and, while keeping your eyes on a fixed spot, gently roll your head from side to side. Observe any differences in the sensation of the support of your left foot on the floor as you roll your head. Can you sense subtle changes in how you balance? Return your right foot to the floor. Rest on the roller.

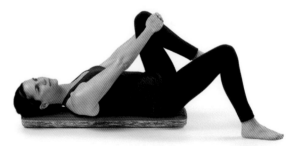

- Slide off slowly and in such a way that you can continue to notice how you do this. Feel how your body is resting on the floor now. Bend your knees and stand your feet on the floor. Feel how your feet are supporting your position. Stand up and observe your posture in standing. Look side to side, seeing if you can sense anything in your feet.

NOTE: As people age, the sensation in the soles of their feet become diminished, and it is very important to facilitate safe learning conditions to support adaptation through the feet that supports upright balance.

Standing **posture and balance** are inextricably linked.
To improve one, you need to address the other. When your back becomes tired
or fatigued after standing, you are most likely overworking in this area.

This section will help you to discover new ways to stand while using less work.

Only try this next idea if your balance on a smooth surface is not already compromised. Remember, it is essential to know your limits and to avoid activities that could be unsafe. Choose the roller surface to stand on that suits your ability. The solid side up has more rocking and the solid side down is more stable. Position yourself near a wall or stable surface for touch support accessibility.

Start with a standing body scan. Notice how your weight is distributed under your feet. Is there more weight towards your heels or your toes? Do you have more weight on one side? Continue to scan your body, noticing each joint, how the two sides compare, your knees, hips and spine, and finally how your head balances on top. Is it difficult to sense certain areas?

- Place the roller towards a wall, leaving enough space between the wall and the roller so your arms can reach out and touch the wall for light support.

- Remove your shoes and stand on the roller with the side that is right for you.

- Start to rock your weight from your heels towards your toes. *Notice what happens as you do this. Do you stop your breathing? What parts of your body do you rely on first? Continue the rocking, but direct the movement to be more from the ankles, letting the rest of your body follow along. Do this several times, making this movement smooth and continuous. Pause on the roller. Return to rocking the roller, but shift your movement to be more from your knees. Allow them to bend and straighten as the roller rocks forward and back. See which movements work together: knees bent/ roller back or vice versa. Gradually reduce the movement to about a quarter of the original movement.*

Notice how your shoulders move with the motion. How does your head respond to the movement? Now, step off the roller and notice how the ground feels. Do you notice a more solid sensation in standing?

movement sequence

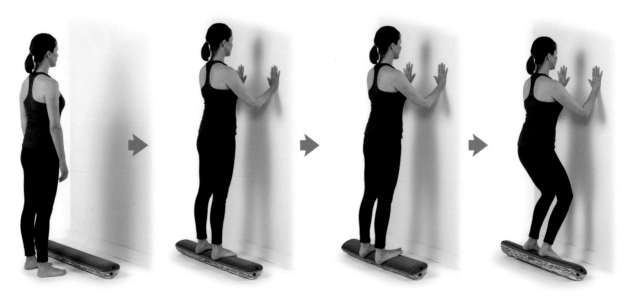

"It is a capital mistake to theorize before one has data."
– Sir Arthur Conan Doyle

- As you stand on the solid floor, place your fingers at the crease of your hips. If you are unsure where this is, lift one leg up and notice where your pants make a crease. This is an approximate location of your hip socket. Most people confuse the hip joint with the bones of the pelvis. (see pelvic clock idea). Can you make this distinction before you move on?

   Return to the roller. With your hands lightly touching the wall for support, crease or bend at the hips to create the rocking movement. How do you do this? Do you squat with this movement or do you bow? Notice how your head is affected with the movement. Repeat this several times. Pause and step off the roller, and stand on the floor to rest.

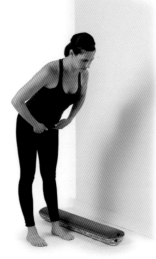

- Reach your hands around to your lower back to touch your spine. Now, round your spine, allowing your bones to stick out into your hands.

   Even though you are only touching one part of the spine, can you think about the full spine as you do this? All 26 spinal bones? When do you breathe in or out with this motion? Lower your hands.

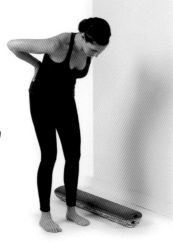

- Now stand on the roller as before, with your hands lightly touching the wall for balance. Start to rock the roller back and forth and remember the earlier movements of your spine. Can you sense these areas moving? Is your head part of your spinal movement? Then pause in the middle.

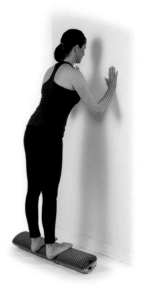

- Still standing on the roller, look down and up. Can you sense how your body accommodates this? Start to let the roller rock with your movement, keeping the head movement small and slow. Can you include all of the prior movements you did while rocking the roller? As you isolate and attend to each part of your movements, it is similar to an orchestra tuning and preparing for a concert. When you organize and put the movements together, they will harmonize with your balance. Repeat this several times and then pause. Step down off the roller and rest.

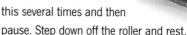

- Notice how you are standing compared to before. Has it changed? Can you sense a change in your posture? Look up and down. Can you feel an adjustment through your whole body? Walk around and see if you can notice the spring in your step, a new softness in your walking.

Now you may begin to create ways to stand for longer periods without experiencing back pain. Just by imagining you are balancing on the roller, you can reduce unwanted body tension when you stand.

Generally, we notice much of our balance in our legs. But, as you noticed before, there are many other balance connections in your body. This next idea will help you create more dynamic stability by again refining your balance in your whole body.

Orient the roller SD (easy) or SU (advanced)

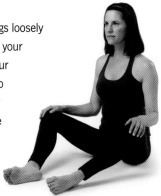

- Sit on the floor with your legs loosely in front of you and feel how your pelvis (bottom) supports your weight. Can you feel the two bones under your buttocks? Does the weight seem to be balanced between these two bones?

- Sit on the roller towards the back so you are able to straddle the roller. Your knees should be bent, your feet on the floor and your hands touching lightly for balance.

- First notice how you balance in this position.

  How long does your body feel from your pelvis to your head? How much work is it to fully lengthen your torso in this position? Allow your hands to rest on the floor or on your legs where they will not interfere with your movements.

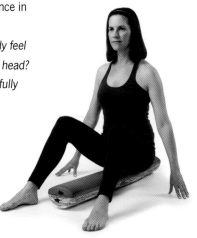

- With your hands lightly touching the floor, start gently tilting the roller a little to each side to notice how you respond to the movement.

  Does your head move, or stay still? Can you notice if it is different from one side to the other? Can you move like this easily? Try and imagine rocking back and forth like riding a horse with an easy gait. Pause in the middle.

- Sit on the roller in the straddle position. Tilt your head slightly side-to-side, allowing your right ear to go towards your right shoulder and your left ear to move towards your left shoulder. Perform a very small movement. Does the roller rock in a particular direction? Start to include the roller a small amount, matching the movement with your head. What do your eyes want to do? After about five to six times, pause in the middle.

  How does your body feel on the roller now? Is it any easier to sit on the roller? Is it easier to breathe?

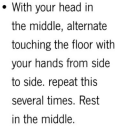

- Return to rocking side-to-side, focus on something in front of you. Can you keep your head in the middle? Can you try to do this without excessive tension? Repeat this five to six times, then pause.

- With your head in the middle, alternate touching the floor with your hands from side to side. repeat this several times. Rest in the middle.

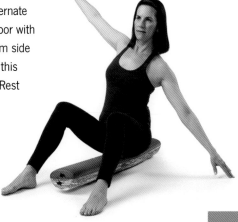

- Gently slide off the roller and feel how your pelvis is resting on the floor now. Can you feel your pelvis more fully?

- Return to the roller and slowly shrug your left shoulder, allowing your body to follow the movement. Notice how you reposition on the roller. Repeat this several times. Try this movement with your right shoulder.
  Which shoulder is easier for you to do?

- Slide off the roller and rest on the floor in sitting. Compare how this feels from before. Notice if there are any changes.

- Sit on the roller and slowly rock your pelvis backward, tucking your tailbone under you. *Notice how this shortens your torso. What does your head do? Continue with the movement, following your breath and observing when you inhale or exhale. Try it with both variations. Shorten and exhale five to six times. Shorten and inhale five to six times. Which is easier?*

- Next, do the opposite movement and lengthen your torso, rolling your pelvis forward and tipping your tailbone back. Allow your back to follow without strain. Gently arch through your full spine. *Notice how this affects your head movement. How do you breathe? Exhale as you arch upward several times, then inhale when you arch upward. Which feels easier? Pause in the middle. Return to tipping the roller side-to-side and observe whether this is easier. (Often when you improve movement in one direction, there is an improvement in other directions).*

- Now, allow your eyes to look upwards. Do you automatically tilt your head upward? Try it first with your eyes only, rolling them upward and then downward. Make the

movement small, smooth and continuous. Be sure not to hold your breath, and make the movements with very little tension in your body. Now start to follow with your head, beginning with your eyes. The movements should be synchronized so they blend into each other. Do this several times and then rest in the middle. Return to rocking the pelvis backward and forward and notice how this has changed following the movement with the eyes.

- Slide off the roller and rest while sitting on the floor.

- Return to the roller in the straddling position. Place your feet one at a time on the roller. When you are ready, lift your arms up to the sides to balance.

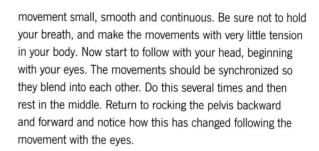

How do you balance? Are you holding your breath? Allow yourself to adjust for your balance, even if you need to touch the floor at times. Experiment with your leg position to capture your balance: knees bent with your legs turned outward or knees bent and pointed towards the sky.

- If you have your balance in this position, look round the room. If you lose your balance, where were you looking?

- Now, return your feet to the floor and slide off the roller. Sit on the floor and notice how weighted your pelvis feels. The easy feeling you notice occurs when your body has become more skeletally organized; meaning, the skeleton is doing the appropriate amount of support. This allows your muscles to be freed and ready for action. Get up and walk around the room. See if it is easier to turn your neck and look behind you. Sit on a chair and notice how easy it is to support your new posture. Notice your length and how your shoulders don't have to tense to help you find this position.

Now that you have played with solving this new balance strategy, see if you can observe how your balance can be more internally monitored—like you observed when you practiced balancing with movement awareness on the roller.

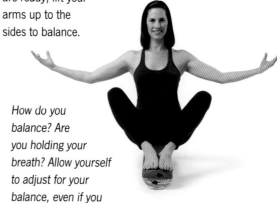

There are many strategies for lengthening your hamstrings.

> Your hamstrings, located at the back of your thighs, are important muscle contributors for upright support. There is evidence that shows you can create conditions to lengthen muscles through active movement and without stretching. Here you will be using movement variations with guided attention to create new ways to lengthen your muscles.

These exercises are best done on a smooth floor to avoid any friction of movement with the roller.

Before you sit on the floor, stand and slowly bend forward as if you wanted to touch your toes. (Only do this if you can do it without pain). What is the easy distance you can go without strain? Where do you feel the resistance?

Now sit on the floor with your legs out long. How does this feel, do you have to lean back to do this? Do your knees pop up from the floor because your hamstrings are shortened? How much distance is there from the back of your knees to the floor?

Orient the roller solid side up: SU

- Sit with your bottom on the roller and your feet on the floor, knees slightly bent. The roller should be positioned as if you are sitting on an unstable bench.

- Bend your knees and place your hands under your left thigh to support your left leg. Start to tilt the roller forward and back. Do this several times in many different ways—from your pelvis, from your ankles, etc.
  As you do this, stay comfortable and allow your breath to be uninterrupted. Repeat this several times.

- Release your hands and rest while you sit on the roller.

- Next, take hold of your right thigh. Your right hand is wrapped around the outside of your right thigh and your left hand should be placed between your legs so you can lace your fingers together to support your leg. Continue the rocking motion and use your whole body. Repeat this several times. Move slowly and smoothly with each movement.
  Notice any changes. Is there a difference between the two legs? Release your hands and rest while you sit on the roller.

- Return to the last position with your hands wrapped around your right thigh. Now, gently and without force, direct your right ear towards your right knee. As you repeat this several times, make very small movements and allow the roller to assist you with the rocking motion-notice how the roller motion can assist you to move.
  Can you move slowly to follow the movement with your breath? Is it easier to breathe out as you bend or to breathe in? Try both ways and note the differences. Pause in the middle.

- Now, direct your left ear towards your right knee, again, allowing the rocking motion of the roller to assist you. Where do you direct your eyes? Repeat this motion several times.

- Pause and rest on the roller.

- Next, direct your nose towards your right knee, allowing for the front of your body to fold in on itself. Again, try this movement while you breathe out and then while you breathe in. How do these patterns of movement compare? Repeat this a few more times, alternating between breathing in and out.

- Now slide off the roller and sit on the floor. Lengthen your two legs and see if they feel any different.

  Does the back of one thigh rest any closer to the floor? Do you sit more under one side of your pelvis?

- Return to sitting on the roller and repeat the same sequence for your left leg. How do the two sides compare?

- Rest on the roller.

- With both your knees bent, take both hands and hold onto your right foot. (If you are unable to reach your foot, you can hold your lower leg-it is important that you do not stretch to do this). Now slide the right foot slightly away from you, allowing your head to move in the direction of your right knee. Slide the right foot back and pause for a moment. Repeat the same movement several times.

- Rest as you sit on the roller.

- Use both hands on your left foot, and now slide your left foot away. Allow the roller to move to assist you. Do this several times.

- Hold your right foot with your right hand and your left foot with your left hand, gently slide your right foot away and back, then slide your left foot away and back. Alternate. Gently bend downward as you move each foot away from you. Be sure to assist your motion with the rocking of the roller. Do this several times with each side.

  Do you breathe in or breathe out as you perform this movement? What happens with the rest of your body as you do the movement?

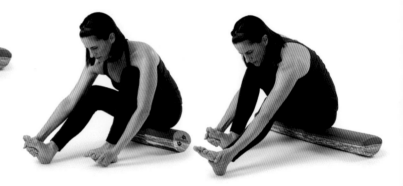

- Slide off the roller to the floor.

- Lengthen your legs out on the floor, and see if this is any easier. Next, stand up and repeat your earlier test by slowly bending forward as if you wanted to touch your toes. Are there any changes? Through attentive guided movements, your body's natural self-correcting system is used. Your muscles naturally become longer since the opposing work is less present to create the unnecessary resistance.

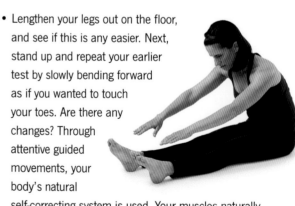

"If you know what you are doing you can do what you want." – Moshe Feldenkrais

TRY THIS:

Take a pair of glasses and fold them up. Do this in as many ways as possible. Once you have exhausted all your ideas, try folding the glasses by fixing one arm of the glasses and move the middle of the glasses to hinge them closed. This may help you think about alternate solutions. We tend to only refer to ways to do things out of long-formed habits, but a shift in perspective may offer a better solution. The release of tight hamstring muscles occurred because the organization of lengthening took place from more than the attachment of your hamstrings.

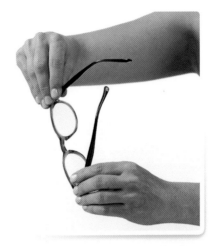

• Research has shown that Feldenkrais lessons can lengthen the hamstrings without stretching. Refer to "Lengthening the Hamstring Muscles Without Stretching Using Awareness Through Movement"-
http://ptjournal.apta.org/content/86/12/1641.full

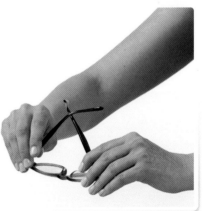

• This sequence can also be done with two links under each sits bone for more variations. See how this compares with the roller. *Do you remember children's pedal cars? Can you see how the pedal action is similar to the reciprocal movement in this idea sequence?*

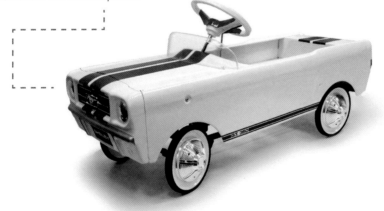

Your spine is connected in a chain-like arrangement composed of twenty-six segments. Through your intelligent nervous system, your spine can either move segmentally or stabilize in parts. Ideally, this spinal action will respond to what your mechanics require. However, because of your daily use and habits, your coordinated spinal movements may become less articulated, spontaneous or effective. What if you could awaken this process by feeling it more clearly in your own body?

This next idea will help you become more aware of your spine and thus help you improve your spinal movement.

start with the body scan
Orient the roller solid side up: SU

- Lie on the roller and allow it to support your head and pelvis. Note the natural curves in your body with the sensation of the roller against your back. Don't do anything with it; don't try to flatten your back or neutralize the curves. Simply notice without doing.

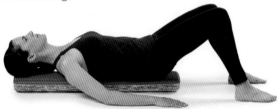

- Next, gently press your feet into the floor to tilt your pelvis and bring your back slightly into the roller. Can you do this without contracting your abdominals? Relax the pressure slowly and allow your pelvis to return to your starting point. Repeat this several times. With each repetition, make the movement smaller and easier. Rest.

    Do you notice the space under your low back more clearly? Can you feel the curves in your spine more prominently?

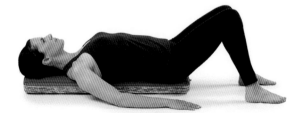

- Gently reverse this movement by tilting the pelvis towards your feet and gently pulling from your legs as if you have suction under your feet.

    Notice how your spine curves into an arch under your low back. Repeat this several times. How do you breathe with this movement?

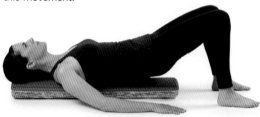

- Next, combine the two movements. Rock your pelvis back and forth, making sure there is no extra effort exerted by any other parts of your body.

    Can you sense any movement in your head? Do you feel equal pressure under your feet when you rock the pelvis? Repeat this several times.

- Rest. Slowly slide off the roller and notice your contact with the floor.

    Is more of your spine now touching the floor?

- Roll to your side and slide back onto the roller. Lying on the roller with your knees bent, bring your feet a little closer to the roller. Press through both feet equally and start to tilt your pelvis, but continue the movement to gently lift your pelvis a little into the air. Continue to make this movement slowly so that you can articulate the lifting of one spinal segment at a time. Only lift your pelvis so that your mid back (ribs) is still touching. Then, lower back down in reverse order. Repeat this step several times. Make certain to not hold your breath or tighten your neck or jaw muscles.

- Rest on the roller.

  Observe how your back is making contact with the roller now. Are there any changes?

- Next, lace your fingers together. Rest them on your belly. Now separate them and re-lace them.

  How do you do this? Does the same finger stay on top each time you lace your fingers together? Next time you put them together, switch them so the opposite hand has the finger on top. What does this feel like? Notice how strange this feels and how habits become comfortable because they are familiar. Continue switching them back and forth several times and then rest your hands on the floor.

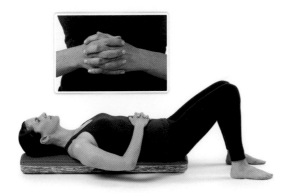

- Lace your fingers together in the original (habitual) way. Slide them under the back of your head, as if to create a hammock to support your head. Now, gently lift your head with your arms as you turn off your neck muscles. Only lift your head about an inch up from the roller and then lower it back down. Repeat this movement slowly, noticing how your spine adjusts to the movement. Are you breathing? Rest, leaving your hands in place.

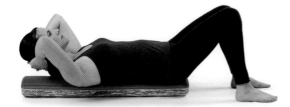

- Again, lift your head gently off the roller—this time a little higher so the spine becomes a little more lifted to about shoulder blade level. Then roll back down, allowing the spine to return in reverse order. Try doing this several times. Position your arms in the best way to support this movement. Try it several ways until you find the easiest way. What happens with your breathing?

  Is it easier to breathe in or out as you lift? Try both.

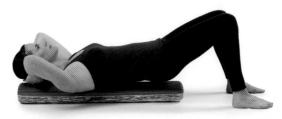

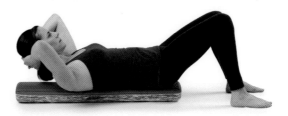

- Rest and gently slide off the roller. Notice your contact with the floor now. Roll to your side and slide back onto the roller.

- Lace your fingers together, this time in the non-habitual way. Place them behind your head and notice how this feels. Now, gently lift your pelvis in the air, articulating the spinal movements one segment at a time and from the bottom on up. As you lower your pelvis, simultaneously lift your head up one segment at a time, top on down. Once you have fully lowered your pelvis, start the movement over, lifting your pelvis as you lower your head and vice versa. Continue rocking up and down your spine several times. Rest.

- Roll off the roller and lower your legs, noticing your contact with the floor.

  What are the changes that you notice? Observe how clear your spine feels to you now.

- Bend your knees and slowly lift your pelvis up off the floor.

  Can you feel your spine more clearly? As you return and rest on the floor, is there a change in the pattern of pressure with your spine?

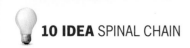

Consider these other ideas:
Switch sides of the roller (solid side down).

Note: Spinous processes (the bony protuberances in the
back of your spine) may be sensitive if they haven't moved like
this in a while. This variation may place too much pressure on
these points. However, if you are looking for less of a balance
challenge, this variation will be more stable. Add a blanket on top
of the curved roller as another option for comfort as you explore
movement variations.

• Another idea: place your feet on the roller as you lie on the
floor. The two sides may be used to note more differences.
If the roller slides or your legs cramp in the back, you might be
generating too much work to lift your spine. An intermediate
step could be to move it up against a wall to keep it from
sliding. This option is an excellent preparation for Pilates work
called 'bird on a perch.'

By exploring these patterns of movement, you help create ways
to integrate new and improved movement patterns with your
everyday movements. You will discover that this set of intentional
movements will be more powerful in improving how you move
than a typical daily exercise routine.

When the **SMARTROLLER** is applied to the front of your body, profound changes may occur in your spine.

This happens through accessing an improved kinesthetic awareness to the front of your body.

If there is any discomfort with this next idea, please apply a small blanket or pad on the roller or start with a rolled-up blanket.

Orient the roller solid side up: SU

Start with a Body Scan. Observe your breathing. Roll onto your front side and feel how your breath compares. Bring yourself to your hands and knees and raise your back up and down, feeling how you do this task. Pay close attention to how your spine moves and if there are any areas where you feel strain.

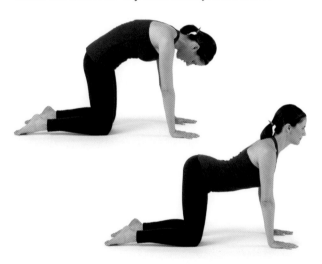

- Place the SMARTROLLER under your body with enough room to rest your forehead on the floor on a rolled towel and place your hands in a push-up position. Start a very small movement to lift your head slightly off the floor, then place it back down. Notice how you do this and where you start the movement. Repeat this several times, reducing your effort with each movement. Rest on the roller.

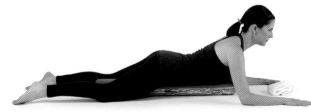

- Bend your knees so your feet are pointed towards the ceiling. Like before, lift your head from the floor. How is the movement different?

  Is it easier or more difficult to perform this movement with your legs bent?

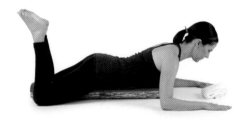

- Come to your hands and knees and rest for a few seconds. Remember that the rests allow time for your brain to discover new ways of moving, so try not to rush through them.

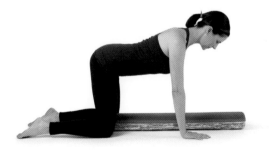

- Return to the roller, with your head resting on the floor, hands in a push-up position and legs stretched out long.

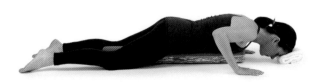

- Now, as your hands are still positioned on the floor, start to pull your right hand slightly away from the floor—without actually breaking contact with the floor. Think of the floor as sticky fly paper and, as you pull with the right arm, notice how this shifts your weight on the roller. Repeat this several times, leaving your forehead in contact with the floor.

    How does your left hand respond? Can you do this without any change in your breathing? Rest in the middle.

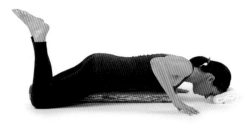

- Repeat this routine with your left hand. Remember to keep reducing the force of the movement.

    How do the two sides compare? Which side seems to move more easily?

- Next, alternate the two sides and allow the roller to rock with you. Observe how this changes the pressure of your chest on the roller. How does the pressure change under your hands on the floor. Can you allow your head to participate? Repeat this several times. Rest.

- Now, press gently into the floor with both hands, then begin to lift both hands. Alternate the two movements back and forth finding a nice slow rhythm. Rest.

- Return to the movement of lifting your head slightly. Is it any easier now? Can you feel how more of your body is involved with the movement?

Remember the
Tai Chi pushing hands reference for how to connect to the floor without imposed force. This allows you to be able to feel through your whole body.

- Rest, and gently slide off the roller and roll onto your back. Have there been any changes? How does your breath feel?

- Return to the roller, head on the floor, hands in push-up position and knees bent. Slowly lift your left knee a small amount up from the floor—just enough to break contact—and lower it back to the floor. Repeat this several times.

    Feel how you distribute your weight as you prepare for this movement. Can you feel how your hands and arms make the adjustments? Pause.

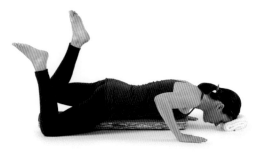

- Repeat the same movement with your right leg. Do the movements several times; notice how it compares to your left leg. Pause.

- Now, lift both knees at the same time, barely raising them off the floor, and take care not to strain your low back. How can you do this so you distribute the weight evenly through your arms, chest, legs, etc.? After you have done this movement a few times, come up to all fours to rest.

- Return to the roller and rest your head on the floor, with your hands in the push-up position and your knees bent. Now, gently push with both hands and start to peel your front side (chest) off the roller slowly as you lower your feet towards the floor. Stop when you reach just below your breast bone (sternum), then roll back down as you bend your knees back. Only go as far as you can go without straining your neck or lifting your belly off the roller. Repeat this movement a few times and then rest on the roller.

    Be sure to breathe throughout the movement. Do you push through your hands equally, or does one hand tend to push harder than the other hand? Can you allow your head to raise with your movement as opposed to lifting your head first?

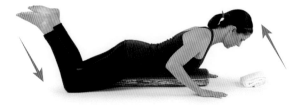

- Rest back on the roller and return to the movement of lifting your head from the floor.
    Has it changed? Is it any easier?

- Now, slide off the roller and roll onto your back, noticing how your body feels.
    What is your contact with the floor like now?

- Without the roller, return to the floor on your hands and knees. Now round your spine and feel for the space on the front of your body that was once resting on the roller. Can you imagine that space closing in on itself? Make this an easy sliding motion and see if you can make the motion uniform.

Imagine this movement on your front side like the movement of two Japanese sliding doors as they close together.

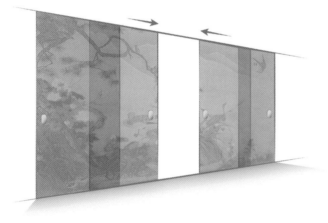

- Now reverse the direction of movement so your chest expands through this space, creating an arch in your low back. Move slowly so you can direct your intention to your front side and feel how this space opens. Create an even distribution of movement where the roller once was. Create the image with this movement like the woman on the front of a ship.

- Next, combine the two movements. See if you can detect how to direct an even distribution of movement throughout your chest and arms. Shift your attention to your spine with your cat-like motions. Notice how shifting your attention to the movement helps create changes. Repeat this while shifting your attention to your front and back.

- Roll onto your back and rest. Notice any changes compared to the beginning. Slowly get up and stand. Notice how three-dimensional your body feels in space. Are you more aware of your entire body now? Often we only think about back problems in our back, but we are three dimensional, and a better sense of awareness to this will help you move in a more dynamic way.

How can you use this idea to help you observe postural strains from tension along the front of your body? Try visualizing how your cat moves while you sit in a chair.

loosening tight hips
IT band alternative

Many people have used foam rollers to massage their outer thigh muscles

and tissues (specifically, the iliotibial band). These superficial tissues are delicate and are also near other sensitive structures such as your femur (thigh bone) and a bursa (a fluid filled sac that aids to lubricate your joints). Fortunately, there are new ways to release this area gently, without pain, while supporting your soft tissue integrity. This next idea will use the floor to create gentle friction to massage your outer hip without the force. You may discover that more than your outer thigh is the cause of the restrictions in your hips.

Orient the roller solid side up: SU
Lie on the floor and perform a Body Scan.

Notice where your feet are pointing. Are there differences between the two sides? Bend your knees and bring your legs together to touch your inner thighs, knees and heels. How easy is this? Lower your legs. Observe where your legs rest.

- Roll onto your left side (this will be the side that you will loosen). Rest your head on your left arm or on a pillow. Place your right hand on the floor with your elbow up in a push-up position. Place your right leg on the roller where your knee and ankle can easily balance and slide your leg back a little with your left leg out long.

   Can you support this position without tensing your body? Adjust yourself until you can easily distribute your weight evenly to balance your leg easily.

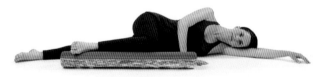

- Positioned like this, roll your whole body slightly forward, towards the floor and back several times. If you need to, readjust the roller to find the best place to allow for this movement.

   As you continue, notice how your body responds. Does your head roll? How do your ribs move? What happens with your left leg, the leg you are lying on, as you move in both directions?

Notice how your leg moves with the contact with the floor. If you move gently, you will see that there is a soft rolling of tissue on your outer left leg. Your body weight will act like a rolling pin.

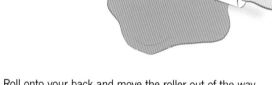

- Roll onto your back and move the roller out of the way. Observe any changes.

- Return to your left side and place your right leg the same way, resting your ankle and knee on the roller. Gently initiate the rocking by pushing with your right hand. See if you can pace the movement with your breath.

   Move slowly, allowing time to notice and intentionally make the movement smoother and continuous. You will soon discover that your entire left side will soften to the floor. Can you sense your spine? Where is your tailbone? Notice how the two legs move. See if you can sense that one leg moves forward while the other moves back. Repeat this several times and then rest on your back.

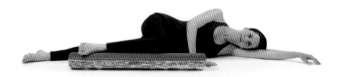

- Return to lie on your left side with your right leg on the roller. Now, straighten your right arm with your palm face down on the floor. Slide your hand away from your body, and notice how your shoulder blade moves. Slide your hand back and repeat this motion several times. As you move, allow your whole body to roll forward in a synchronized manner—as if it's spiraling from the top on down as you move like this. Through this movement, you will allow your tissues to also internally rotate with the floor friction. Pause in the middle.

    Roll onto your back and notice the differences between the two sides. Bend your knees and bring them together. How has this changed? How are your two sides different?

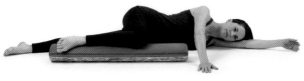

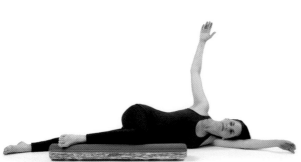

- Repeat this movement on your opposite side. Lie on your right side and place your left leg on the roller. Place your left hand in a push-up position. Repeat the same steps on this side, but move to only 10 percent of your range that you moved on the opposite side. Repeat each step and then roll onto your back and rest.

    Notice how the two sides compare. Now are they more even?

- Bend your knees and stand with your feet on the floor. Bring your legs together so your inner thighs are touching. If you cannot do this, place a pillow between your legs to keep them in contact with each other. Now, take the roller, hold it at the ends and lift it up in front of you. Your arms should be positioned straight up and perpendicular to your body. Without bending your elbows, tilt the roller a little to the right and left. The amount of movement may be small and requires you to keep your legs together. Repeat this several times, reducing the amount of movement with each repetition.

    Observe how your ribs turn and how your full body responds to the movement. How do your ribs and outer thighs relate? Often your outer thighs become over-active from poor turning in your trunk. When you allow for more areas to be involved, it will reduce habitual overwork of these muscles. Rest your arms down, move the roller out of the way and lower your legs. Notice how your legs feel now. Slide them together and see if this has become any easier.

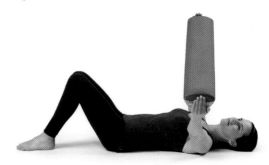

- Slowly roll to your side and stand. See if you notice if your feet are in a different position—maybe closer together? Farther apart? Walk around and feel how your feet make contact with the floor. Do you notice greater ease in taking your steps? What are your footprints like? If you are prone to rolling inward or outward on your feet, you might feel a change in how your feet are touching the ground.

By discovering how you reduced the tension in your hips, you might become more aware of habits that contribute to creating it. You might find that there is an association to tightening your chest, holding your shoulder blades rigid, or many other antagonistic patterns of movement.

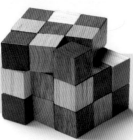

LINKS

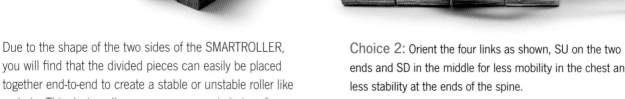

Due to the shape of the two sides of the SMARTROLLER, you will find that the divided pieces can easily be placed together end-to-end to create a stable or unstable roller like a chain. This design allows more movement choices for you to select from. These pieces are called SMARTROLLER LINKS—like links in a chain or a pointer to a site—and they can be used in many applications. Because of the shape, they do not need to be conjoined together. In fact, the way they can connect together is the uniqueness of their design.

Added to your SMARTROLLER, the LINKS allow you to build a longer and even more dynamic roller. By varying the orientation and shape of the LINKS, you will allow for a wide range of possibilities. The solid side up (SU) will help you access more movement, and the solid side down (SD) will allow you to design more stability. The links may also be easier to apply to equipment, such as a Pilates reformer, or with other apparatuses.

Here are a few ideas to get you started, but you can also create your own puzzle variations to find more applications for motor learning. Decide before you put them together what and where you would like to create to heighten movement awareness and performance. Once you have made your playful choices, begin.

Start with the Body Scan. Later, return to the scan to notice any changes in your body positioning. Remember, by drawing attention to differences, you allow for learning through comparison.

Choice 1: Orient the full roller solid side down (SD) and orient one link at the end with the solid side up (SU) for a stable torso and a mobile neck version. The reverse will create less head and neck movement and more torso movement. If it is difficult to rest your head flat on the roller because your head is too far forward, place a foam pad under a link so your head may rest with better contact to avoid strain.

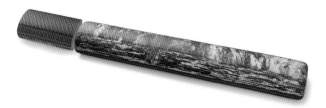

Choice 2: Orient the four links as shown, SU on the two ends and SD in the middle for less mobility in the chest and less stability at the ends of the spine.

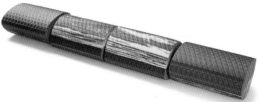

Choice 3: Orient the links as shown to immobilize your upper body with pelvic instability or vice versa. Mix the variations up – the dynamic roller becomes a Rubik's cube. If you are working with children, a fun game to play with them is to have them roll to their side while you change the orientation of the links so they will have to sense the varying orientation. This discovery game is a good way to work with children's posture.

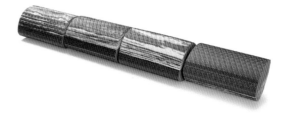

Choice 4: Aligning all the pieces with the same side up is another way to create the experience of sensing where the parts separate. While rocking, see if you are able to discriminate where the parts divide.

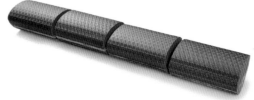

• You can stand on two links to create more variations for standing balance. They can be the same or different, depending on how you are playing with balance. Have your kids stand on the links, as they are engaged with activities that would normally keep them inactive.

• Through playing with the LINKS, can you start to see how your spine can move between stability and mobility depending on your need? Once you discover this dynamic action of your spine, see if you can draw on this awareness in other postural configurations.

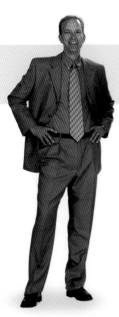
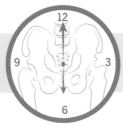

Most people, when asked to touch their hips, **will actually touch their pelvis.**

The pelvis (Latin word for basin) is the largest bone in the body and is often associated with your core muscles. The hip is a joint, made between your femur (thigh bone) and pelvis. This distinction is important, since how you think about your body and how you sense your body are connected. This next idea will help you coordinate new movements that help in all activities, especially with sports training and preparation for pregnancy.

start with the body scan

Orient the roller solid side up (SU) and orient a LINK solid side up (SU). Place the LINK perpendicular to the end of the roller, almost touching to allow a rocking motion. (Rock the link a few times to note the action.)

• Lie on the roller as shown, but slide down to rest your pelvis off the end, on top of the SR link. If you can easily rock the link up and down, you are in the right place.

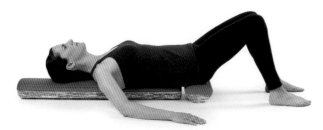

• With your knees bent, position your legs where you can balance easily. Try a few variations to find your best choice. Remember to rest off the roller anytime you need to.

Pay attention to your breathing and your contact with the roller. Notice how your spine touches in some places and where it does not touch. See if you can notice the natural curves in your back.

Imagine there is a clock under your pelvis (roughly where you have placed the LINK). The face of the clock is oriented with 12:00 pointed towards your head, 6:00 at your tail bone, 9:00 off to the right hip and 3:00 towards your left hip. Gently press into the floor with both feet to tilt your pelvis towards 12:00 on your pelvic clock. Repeat this several times. This pelvic tilting movement may feel like an exercise you have done before, but

see if you can approach it differently. The following prompts will guide you to access new potent movements.

Remember to apply a very gentle pressure to allow the motion to move through your whole body. See if there is a gentle motion that connects to your head. Does your head move to the motion? Rest.

• Gently rock the pelvis in the opposite direction as if your feet have suction and you are lightly pulling with your legs to roll the pelvis towards the 6:00 on your pelvic clock. Your feet should not break contact with the floor. This movement guides you through an alternate way of arching your back with less of the arching directed from your back muscles.

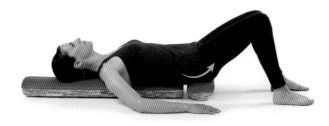

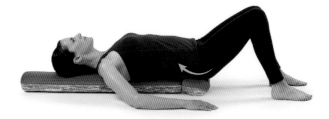

Which directional movement was easier to accomplish: 12:00 or 6:00? Repeat this movement a few times and slowly add both directions to allow the roller LINK to act as a teeter-totter. Can you feel what is happening with your head? If there was a similar clock under your head, do the movements relate to each other? Rest.

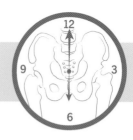

* Improving rhythmical motion of your pelvis will not only help with sexual or playful movements, but will also help reduce and absorb ground forces through your skeleton. When working properly, your skeleton has a spring-like action that allows transmission of force to move through you.

Extend your left leg and continue to rock your pelvis gently by pressing into the floor and releasing.

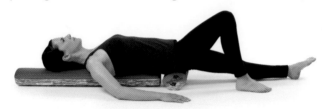

What direction does this correspond to your pelvic clock? 1:00? 2:00? Repeat this motion several times, allowing for the movement to travel through your body. Is your head moving? In which direction does it move? Bring your right leg back up and rest.

- Repeat these steps with your right leg.

What direction does your pelvis move now? 11:00? 10:00? Repeat this motion several times following the movement in your whole body. Is this easier or more difficult? Bend your left leg back up and rest.

- Slowly lift your pelvis up and turn the roller link to be in line with the SMARTROLLER without touching them together. Rest your pelvis back down.

- Next, keeping your foot in contact with the floor, gently tilt your right foot outward to roll your ankle outward. Allow your right knee to follow. Roll your foot back and repeat this wobble action a few times.

  As you do this, feel if your pelvis tilts to the right. Does it move directly towards 3:00 or slightly off? Is there any movement in your head? Repeat this several times, making it lighter, easier and without interrupting your breathing. Can you separate the movement from your breathing? Rest in the middle.

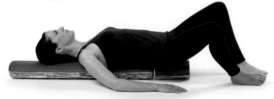

- Repeat this set with your left foot. Allow for your left leg to follow, and wobble it to the left and back.
  Is this movement easier to do on this side or on your right?

Does the pelvis roll directly towards the 9:00 position? How does your head respond? Continue the movement but reduce the intensity to half the previous range of motion and then reduce it in half again. Continue this process until the movement is hardly detectable. Pause in the middle and rest.

- Roll gently to the floor while sliding both rollers away and lie on your back. Try making this transition smoothly and fluidly.

- Bend your knees. Redefining the points of your pelvic clock, gently repeat the movements of pressing into the floor to tilt your pelvis to 12:00 and 6:00. Follow this movement by tilting your pelvis right and left to orient towards 3 and 9 o'clock. Rest.

- Start the movement of tilting towards 12:00, gently tilting your pelvis to the right and allowing for the pelvis to arc in a clockwise motion. Continue on down connecting each number on the clock.

  Notice if all the clock numbers are connected. Which numbers are missing? Pay attention to the rest of your body when you jump over a number. This may help you discover new ways to coordinate missing movements that might have gone unnoticed before. Rest. Lower your legs down. Does your body feel differently on one side compared to the other?

- Bend your knees. Reverse the movement so now you are moving counterclockwise. How does this movement compare? Which areas are less clear? More clear? Rest. Notice your contact with the floor compared to the beginning. Is your back resting more fully?

- Roll to your side and come to sitting and then standing. Walk around sensing your pelvis in space. Follow with a familiar exercise program and see if you are able to attend to your pelvic clock.

Through these movement variations you may discover and solve for yourself a new way to integrate your pelvic movements, allowing you to not only move smarter but to help you feel stronger. When you watch sports with this new understanding, see how skilled athletes use their bodies in this coordinated way. Our brains possess what is called the mirror neuron system. Watching skilled movements after you are familiar with the same movements can help increase your clarity to improve performance. "Slowly you will become aware of a strange sensation, unfamiliar to most people: a clearer picture of your self-image." – M. Feldenkrais

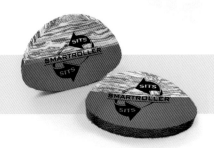

Sitting for long periods can be a challenge.

There are many ergonomic chairs and environmental set-ups that can support your sitting position. However, research has shown that many challenges of prolonged sitting are directly related to posture. Did you know that a skeleton can sit unsupported with minimal muscle support? "Ideally, the weight of your body should be balanced on your skeleton. The primary role of your muscles should be to align your skeleton to provide that balanced support."[1] However, the confusion arises when we think of this as a fixed-static position.

Physical therapists and most movement educators agree that a good way to attain good posture is to balance your weight on your sits bones, the bottom of your pelvis. We don't often think of sitting on our seats as a balancing skill, but every move we make—e.g., turning our heads, shifting in our seats to reach or even breathing—requires a new adjusted balance position. "When you feel grounded and supported by the surface beneath you, your upper body can relax and center itself over the base that your lower body provides. When you don't feel supported from below, you tense your upper body in an attempt to make up for that lack of support."[2] Mabel Todd, anatomist, educator, and author of the *Thinking Body*, often referred to this form of support as "structural hygiene".[3] Muscles are not designed to do the work of the bones and can lead to what Feldenkrais called "cross motivation between muscles" – that is, a rigid and tight posture. Posture is dynamic, and the SITS are kinesthetic learning tools or tactile aides designed to help you do this more easily.

The following idea will help you find your good dynamic posture.

- Start with a sitting body scan. Sit on the edge of a firm chair with both feet on the ground and notice how you are sitting. Can you feel the sits bones of your pelvis? Is the weight evenly placed between the two sits bones? Does your head feel slightly forward or directly over your shoulders? What is your breathing like?

- Now, look up and down taking note of how easy it is to do this. Is there any strain in this movement?

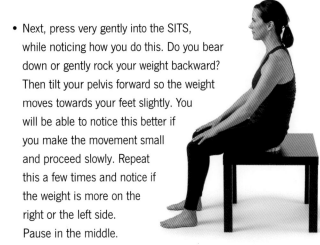

- Slightly lift one buttock and place one SITS pad under one sits bone and then the other. The SITS should be slightly visible from behind to create a wedge, much like a heel insert. Observe how this shifts you slightly forward. Is there any change in how your head is positioned?

- Next, press very gently into the SITS, while noticing how you do this. Do you bear down or gently rock your weight backward? Then tilt your pelvis forward so the weight moves towards your feet slightly. You will be able to notice this better if you make the movement small and proceed slowly. Repeat this a few times and notice if the weight is more on the right or the left side. Pause in the middle.

- Look up, then down. Repeat this several times, noticing what happens when you rock forward on the SITS and when you rock back. How does it correlate to your head movement? Pause in the middle.

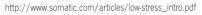

[1] http://www.somatic.com/articles/low-stress_intro.pdf
[2] http://www.somatic.com/articles/low-stress_intro.pdf
[3] Todd, M. THE THINKING BODY

- Now, lift the balls of your feet from the floor, leaving your heels down. Does this cause any movement in your pelvis? Do you shift forward or back as you do this? Next, tilt your weight onto your toes, lifting your heels. How does this affect your position on the SITS? Pause in the middle. Now alternate the movements, shifting your weight to your toes then your heels. Repeat this a few times. Think of the movement as if you are a child on a swing as you allow yourself to rock back and forth.

- Remove the SITS. Notice what has changed. Can you feel your four point skeletal balance more easily? Look up and see if this movement has improved? Does your weight shift in your four-point position? How has this newly acquired awareness of your sits bones affected your sitting?

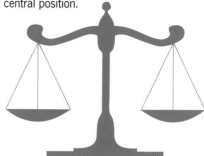

Now that you have this awareness, see if you can imagine your own sits bones several times a day. What shifts in your sitting as you do this? You may now notice when you prepare to get out of your chair that you can feel your weight transfer from your sits bones towards your feet to get up. This ergonomic way to stand up will help you use better body mechanics while you improve strength in more optimal muscles to transition to standing.

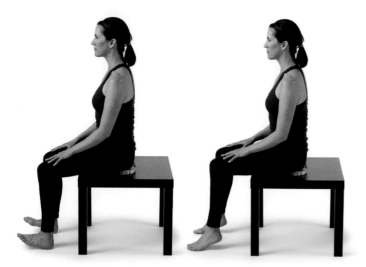

We all prefer to sit on one sits bone more than the other and we are not usually aware of this. The SITS provide just the right internal feedback to align your pelvis to a more balanced position. Think of it as a scale, allowing for you to organize better balance in a central position.

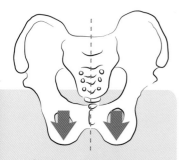

Sits bones, like their name implies, are the bony 'heels' of your pelvis, well designed to support your body weight. When you sit on a bicycle seat, you are sitting on these bones.

When you are unaware of sitting unevenly on your sits bones, your spine can develop compensatory curves. Over time, this creates strains and pains in many places.

This idea will help you reduce or diminish an uneven spinal curve to allow you to find a better support in sitting.

Sit on a firm chair to do these next movement sequences. You can modify them if you are sitting on the floor. Scan your posture as you sit. Notice the weight under your pelvis or under your buttocks. Are you weighted on one sit bone more than the other? How do you notice this? Feel how your weight is in your feet. Are both heels touching the floor? Would you need to adjust your position to stand up, or are you in a ready posture with your weight evenly balanced on your feet? How are you breathing? Can you feel your breath in your abdomen, chest, sides and back?

Now look to your right, and see how far you can turn. Mark the last thing you see without strain. Next, turn to the left. Measure this as well.

- Now place the SITS under your sits bones. Start with orienting the SITS as shown in the picture. The placement does not need to be exact-you can estimate this position. As long as the SITS are matched alike, the orientation is less important.

- In this position, feel how the two sides compare. Are both your shoulders level? If you are not sure, drop your hands to your sides and feel for which arm seems longer.

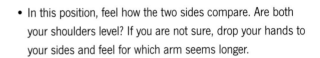

- Which SITS do you have more pressure on? Remove the SITS from the side with the most weight. Feel how this shifts the balance in your body. Gently roll your pelvis forward and back. Notice the sensation of your uneven sit position. Can you follow this through your whole body? Repeat this several times to allow you to sense the uneven movement of your pelvis—how your ribs bend unevenly and if there are any changes in how your head moves. Pause.

- Next, lift the arm on the side that you have the SITS under (if you have the single SITS under your left side, lift your left arm and vice versa). Place this hand on your head with your elbow in the air. Gently tilt your head a little to that same side and back. Make sure you don't just bend at the neck, but, instead, bend through your whole trunk.

- Repeat this movement several times, breathing out as you bend and in as you return back in position. Rest with your arm down for a moment.

- With the same hand, reach across to touch and hold your opposite shoulder. On this same side, slide your heel away so your leg is straight.

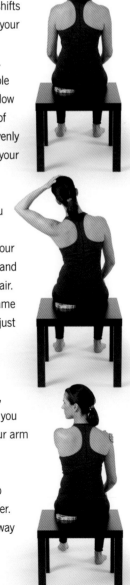

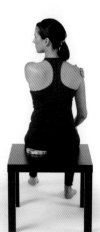

- Gently turn your body towards the side where the SITS are positioned as you guide your shoulder with your hand. Let your head and eyes turn in the same direction.

- Continue to turn like this and add lengthening to your straight leg. You should be turning with your whole body now, but reduce the turn to half the movement with which you started.

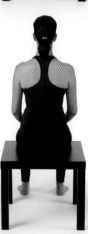

- Return to the middle. Remove the SITS and see how you are sitting now. Are you more balanced? Look from side to side and see how it feels to look in the two directions.

- Do you notice it is easier to turn to one side?

- Now repeat the whole sequence for the opposite side to see how they compare.

- When you notice you are slightly stiff in turning your head, start to shift your weight from one sits bone and find the side that supports the better movement. This will help you discover how this process works beyond simple exercises. You will use your natural problem solving skills to improve how you move.

The preceding ideas helped you improve your strength through better alignment, organization and reduced muscular resistance. These next ideas will help introduce new ways to use resistance exercises while adopting this form of sensory motor learning. Effective strength also possesses reversibility. Meaning, refined and controlled movement can reverse direction at any time in the range. See if your movement precision will allow for you to do this.

The first time you do each sequence, carry out the movements slowly without the resistance. Once this is done, add the resistance with more attention to performing the movements more smoothly and without compromising the quality.

Start with the Body Scan. Scan in sitting, standing or lying position, depending on the position the exercise requires. Our props used are the three to four pound weighted balls, the BodyBlade®, resistance band and the Pilates ring. Try the LINKS for substitutions and for variations. (Also see LINKS and SITS with strength addressed separately.)

Orient the roller solid side up (SU) or down (SD)

① SCAPULAR CONTROL:
SD | prop: soft weights
This exercise is best done following Shoulder Opener Idea to refine your upper body strength.

- Lie on the roller letting the roller support your head and pelvis. Hold two weighted balls and bring them in towards your chest. Weighted balls are preferred because of their shape to reduce wrist strain. Attend to where you have placed your feet and to the distribution of pressure under both of your feet.

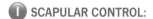

- Raise the balls out in front of you towards the ceiling. Are both arms lined up? Does one feel longer than the other?

- Slowly open your arms to the sides while tracking the movement throughout your body. Do not go beyond a 45-degree angle from the floor to avoid strain in your shoulder joints. Allow your shoulder blades to move at the same time and distance. Return your arms back to the starting position. Repeat this motion ten times.

  Notice the differences between the two arms. Where are the movements smooth and continuous? Where does the movement have a jerky sensation? Is your breath continuous? As you repeat the movement, follow your arms with your peripheral vision. Rest, placing the balls close to your chest.

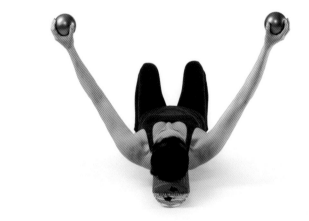

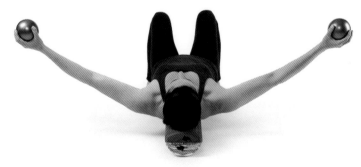

- Next, return your arms up in the air, 90 degrees from your body. Slowly open only your right arm to the side to about 45 degrees. Can you feel how your body adjusts to this asymmetrical position? Feel how your feet respond. Do you feel more grounded? What happens in your chest and upper back to support this movement? Repeat this movement ten times and then open your left arm ten times to compare.

  Return the balls to the floor. Finish by gently rocking back and forth then slowly rolling off the roller.

> "Hold everything as if it was made of glass,
> but grasp everything as if it was made of stone." – Daniel Barrows

⚋ SHOULDER STRENGTH—FRANKENSTEIN ARMS:
SU | prop: soft weights
This exercise is to improve your upper body strength with coordinated core control.

• Lie on the roller supporting your head and pelvis.

• Take two weighted balls and bring them into your chest. Lift them up in the air like the scapular control exercise. This time, allow for a small gap between the two balls. Move the balls only as far as you can reach without moving your shoulder blades forward. Approximate this movement—don't worry if you are unsure if this is correct. The value in the exercise is the focused attention to how you refine your movement coordination.

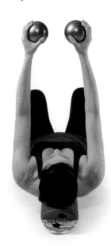

• Lengthen only your right arm towards the ceiling, allowing the roller to roll with the movement. Avoid bending your elbows. Slowly return to your original position. Repeat this five times, making the movement smoother and more fluid.

By keeping your elbows from bending, you will heighten your sensitivity to your shoulder blades to support coordination in this area. Do this smoothly and in one continuous motion. Pause in the middle. Repeat this five times for your left arm.

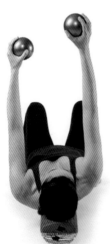

• How do both arms compare? Return to the middle and lower your arms towards your chest and pause.

• Return your arms to the ceiling, and alternate the reach movement five to six times with each arm, making the movement smoother with each new repetition. Pause.

• Lift both arms towards the ceiling. Lengthen you right arm and, as you slowly lower your right arm, start to open your right arm out to the side to the floor. Move only to about 45 degrees from the floor and return.

Notice if there is any change from when you performed this test for the scapular control exercise. Feel how your spine readjusts while you stabilize your body. Repeat this movement five times and then pause in the middle.

• Repeat this exercise with your left arm. Notice any differences between the two.

⚋ DIAPHRAGM FOR CORE CONTROL— Exercise band around the ribs:
SU (beginner), SD (advanced) | prop: resistance band
This exercise will help you create better sensitivity in your upper body and help you integrate your arms with your full body and core connections. Core control is essential for full body conditioning and strength. How you sense your core relationships and integrate it into your self-image may be the missing ingredient in accessing your true strength.
Please review the safety instructions for resistance bands before you proceed with this next exercise.

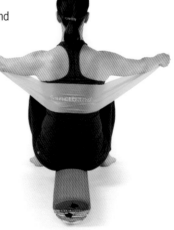

• Sit at the end of the roller and place the resistance band against your back at shoulder blade level with the ends wrapped around to the front. Reach with your right hand for the left band and your left hand for the right band. This creates a crisscross pattern in front.

• Hold the band in one hand as you to lower yourself on the roller. Allow the roller to support your head and pelvis, and keep your knees bent. Take hold of your band with both hands in the criss-cross pattern described above. Lower your elbows so you can rest them on the floor. Pause in this position to notice how your breathing feels with the resistance.

Can you feel the front, back and sides of your ribs equally? What areas do you feel more prominently? Try not to over grip the band with your hands.

- Lift your right hand and extend your elbow as you pull the band diagonally to the right in an approximately 45-degree angle. Orient your hand and wrist in this direction to avoid strain. Repeat this movement five times with the right arm only. Notice how your shoulder blade feels with the roller against your back. How does your body react to your balance and the asymmetrical pull? Can you breathe continuously and avoid excess tension in your jaw and face?

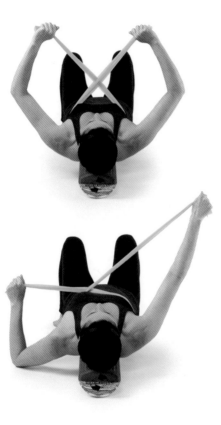

- Repeat this exercise with your left arm five times. Compare this with your right side; how are they different? How do you breathe while you move with this side? Pause, lowering both arms to the floor.

- Now, pull both arms away at the same time. Do this slowly to see if you use them equally or if one dominates over the other. Repeat this five times.

- Bring the band back; release the band gently to rest your arms and roll to the floor. Notice how your low chest feels. Follow with some standing upper body weights and note whether you have a stronger connection to your chest after this preparation.

IV CORE CONTROL—Exercise band around pelvis:
SU | prop: resistance band

This exercise will prepare you for the following exercise: pelvic floor control (the internal working of your pelvic muscles). Wrap your resistance band around your abdomen, reaching the ends towards the back of your pelvis and criss-crossing them back to the front. Tuck the ends in. In this configuration, lie on the band on your roller. Place your hands on your lower ribs to sense how your ribs respond to these guided prompts.

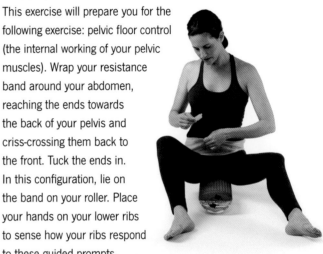

- With this arrangement, lie on your roller to support your head and pelvis and keep your knees bent. Notice how you breathe with the band wrapped around your lower abdomen.

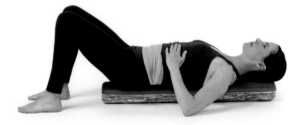

- Follow your breath and start to exaggerate the movement in your belly. Do this for about five breaths.
  Attend to how your chest moves with this exaggerated breath. The band will help you to sense your lower trunk in a three-dimensional way. Return to normal breathing and notice how it compares.

- Next, breathe out with quick bursts of breaths. Observe what muscles you use for this. Continue this way for five more breaths. Return to normal breathing.

- Breathe in quick bursts of breaths, noticing how this feels. Repeat the breathing pattern five times and then rest.

- Next, alternate between breathing with five quick breaths in and then five quick breaths out. Pause.

- Roll to the floor gently and remove the band. Notice how your lower abdomen feels.

"Powerful movement is created if the whole system of muscles, bones and other tissue works together in a coordinated way." – Eric Franklin

V PELVIC FLOOR CONTROL:

SD | prop: Pilates ring or medium size firm ball

- Lie on your back, resting your head and pelvis on the roller. Your knees are bent. Place the Pilates ring between your legs around mid thigh.

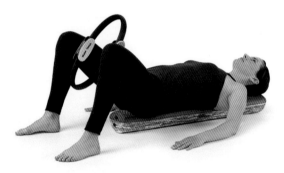

Drawing on the former exercise, notice your breathing. Think about the space between your navel and your pubic bone. The roller will help you notice pressure on your sacrum, which frames the back of your pelvis.

- Now, think of the Pilates ring as a metaphor for the internal ring of muscles in between your legs and gently squeeze the ring while you draw your muscles upward inside your perineal area (groin).

  Try to not over do this so you can sense what muscles you are contracting. Can you do this without holding your breath? Repeat this 5 times, making sure you relax between each repetition. Pause.

- Return to squeezing the ring in quick bursts. Notice how your lower abdomen feels during this action. Continue to do this exercise as you release any unwanted tension in your body. Repeat this five times and rest. Remove the ring and gently rock back and forth on the roller to reduce any unnecessary tightness. This will prepare you for the next core control exercises or your own core exercise.

VI ABDOMINALS: With both knees in table-top position, start with SD and then progress to SU. This exercise is ideally performed after the Single-Leg balance Idea and will help you create more dynamic core control.

- Lie on the roller with either the SU or SD. Find the easiest place to balance and slowly lift one leg at a time to table-top position (hips positioned 90 degrees from your torso). Reduce tension throughout your body while you engage your lower abdomen.

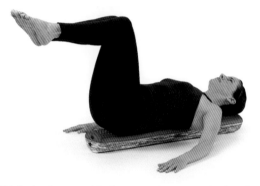

Think about your pelvic floor muscles as you do this. Can you quiet your movement so you can balance in the middle without rigidity? As you reduce unwanted tension, balancing should become easier and will help you directly engage your lower trunk.

- Lower your legs and pause.

- Return your legs to the table–top position and slowly lift your hands so just your finger-tips touch the floor. Start to explore this balance through your trunk. The SMARTROLLER provides you with a wobble board to challenge your core connection. Maintain this position as long as you can hold it with precision and core control. Try not to confuse strain for good muscular engagement. Lower your feet to the floor one at a time and rest.

- Return your legs to the table–top position and slowly roll your head from side to side, tracking with your eyes first, and then follow the movement with your head.

  Sense how your body responds to your head and eye movements. Are you able to sense your balance from your pelvic center?

- Lower your feet to the floor and pause. Rock gently back and forth and slide off the roller. Stand up and walk around.

Ⅶ ABDOMINALS 2—Partial curl ups:
SD, SU | prop: soft weight
Before you do sit-ups with your former habits, consider doing this next sequence of movements with an improved body awareness.

- Lie on the roller with SD first, then proceed to SU. Hold a weight of about three to five pounds in both hands (depending on your skill and control level).

- Lift the weight up to the sky, creating a triangular shape with your arms. Watching it with your eyes, lift the weight overhead, performing this movement mindfully. Lower the weight towards your hips as you lift your head slowly. See if you can do the movement while you think of lengthening your spine. Return the weight overhead as you lower your spine, segment by segment back to the roller. This reverse direction requires good eccentric control (lengthening contraction). Eccentric control is often used for functional conditioning because it is more prominent with our complex daily actions.

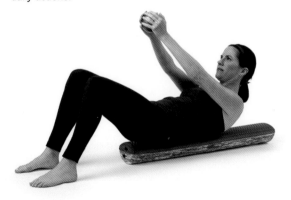

Repeat this exercise five to six times. Feel how you connect to your balance through your feet. Note: Often abdominal work does not allow you to draw on the connection to your skeletal support for stability. This will help prompt grounding of your feet to the floor. Through connecting to the subtleties of balance, you can learn to draw on this sensation for good spinal control when you need to lift heavy objects. With practice, learners begin to pay more attention to relevant feedback information through motor learning (motor learning concepts, Schmidt and Wrisberg, 2008).

- Lift the arms directly up towards the ceiling. Move the arms together to the right without deforming the triangle and feel the connection to the oblique muscles (diagonal abdominal muscles) and your trunk. Next, tilt your arms over to the left. Perform this movement five to six times and pause in the middle.

- Lift your arms up towards the ceiling. Now, start the partial sit-up but direct your hands towards your left knee, creating a slight diagonal twist in that direction.
  Notice the point of contact to the roller as you roll up. Where are you directing your eyes? As you lower back down, notice how you are performing this motion. When do you breathe in or out?

- Repeat this exercise with the other side and compare the two sides. Return to doing the exercise with the weight in the center and see if this has changed. Lower the weight to the floor and gently rock side to side and roll off.

Ⅷ FULL BODY STRENGTHENING: *prop:* BodyBlade®
This variation is similar to the weighted ball exercises but will be substituted with the BodyBlade, a unique training tool. The BodyBlade will add a vibratory action which will boost your muscular engagement through your core elements and allow you to do more coordinated progressions. The action equally opposing the destabilizing forces produced by the BodyBlade helps create more integrated connections throughout your whole body. Almost anything you do with a free weight can be done with the BodyBlade.

- Lie on the roller SD (easy) or SU (advanced), with your knees bent. Hold your BodyBlade with both hands. Follow the partial sit-up routine, substituting the BodyBlade.

- Next, sit on the end of the roller. Start to roll back and pause half way down to about a 45-degree angle. While keeping your spine long, start shaking or driving the BodyBlade. Sustain this vibratory action without compromising your position.

Can you sense your inner abdomen with this exercise? See if you can maintain stability without becoming rigid. If you hold your breath, you most likely will be bracing muscles that interfere with your intended core muscles. Stop driving the BodyBlade and roll back up to rest.

- Sitting straight up, begin driving or oscillating the BodyBlade oriented horizontally in the wide position again. Roll half way down as before and pause. Lift your arms towards the ceiling so the BodyBlade is now oriented horizontally overhead and the motion is up and down. See if you can sustain the same length as before for 30 seconds, then lower your arms in front and return to your start position.

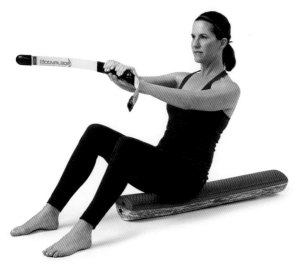

- Come back to sitting, repeat the partial roll down and twist to your right. In this position, begin driving the BodyBlade again and sustain this for about 30 seconds. Return to the middle.

  Where are you directing your eyes? Is your head in the direction in which you are pointing the BodyBlade? Can you center your head in between the direction of both your arms?

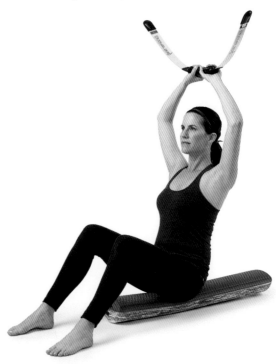

- Place the BodyBlade on the floor and roll down onto the roller. Rock back and forth, and roll off the roller to the floor.

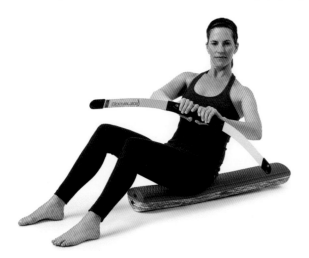

- Follow these steps with the opposite side for 30 seconds and then sit back up.

  Is this side more organized? More controlled? More difficult?

(IX) CORE STRENGTH—Bridge:

SD (beginner), SU (advanced)
This exercise will address pelvic control through balance and is best done after the Spinal Chain Idea.

- Lie on your back, resting your head and pelvis on the roller. Slowly lift your pelvis up and roll your spine upward in sequential order. Then, roll your spine back down.

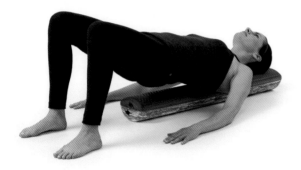

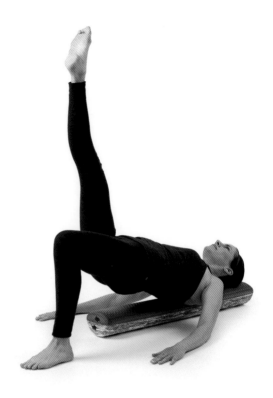

- Return to the same position, but see if you can rest with your pelvis in the air.

  How level is your pelvis? If one side is lower, try lowering the other side to match it. Then return to making the other side higher. Do this a few times so you can feel what is involved in the movement, then lower all the way back down.

- Return to the same position and roll your pelvis up in the air. Slowly straighten your left leg out away from you.

  How do you adjust to this movement? Can you stabilize your whole body, without stiffening? Lift your left leg a little higher and return it back down, slowly bending your knee to place your foot to the ground. Roll your spine back down and pause.

- Roll your pelvis in the air. Slowly straighten your right leg out, away from you.

  How does the movement compare with this side? Lift your right leg a little higher and return it back down, while bending your knee and placing your foot on the ground. Roll your spine back down and pause.

- Return to the same position and roll your pelvis in the air. Slowly straighten your right leg out, away from you. Hold this position and lower your spine to the roller. Notice how you do this with only one leg for support and repeat this exercise with the opposite side.

  Gently rock back and forth, and slowly roll to the floor. Observe your contact with the floor; roll to your side, stand up and walk around.

Ⓧ **ROLL UP TO SIT:** SU; this exercise will help you incorporate balance and core recruitment in a more challenging way. You will also be able to discover what happens when you are performing a more difficult exercise. See if you can keep a playful attitude as the movements become more difficult.

• Lie on your back, resting your head and pelvis on the roller.

• Lift your right leg and hold it with both hands laced together underneath your right thigh. Hold your legs with your arms relaxed as if your arms form a hammock support for your legs. Your left foot remains in contact with the floor. (Note: it is important for your arms to be relaxed and long throughout all these movements to insure that your core muscles are working, not your arm muscles.)

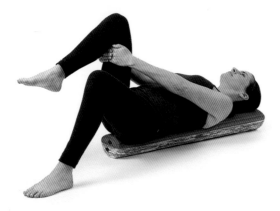

• In the easiest way possible, roll up to sitting. Be sure to not bend your arms or hold your breath while you balance on the roller.

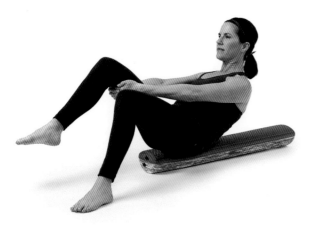

• Roll back down onto the roller in the reverse pattern, noticing how you do this. If you fall off the roller, play with it and be sure to do it in a way that you may learn from it.

• Once you have experimented with this a few times, try this with your left leg and notice how you do it. How do your legs compare? Is one side more successful?

• Place the roller to the side for a moment. Repeat your original movement and hold your right leg with both hands to roll up to sit.

• Can you simplify the movement? See if you can reduce your effort and breathe easily. Try to stop and start the movement. Pause.

• Repeat the movement, but, this time, imagine you are on the roller.

• Notice how the pressure changes along your back, pelvis, and ribs. How does your other leg respond to the movement? Try reversing the start position to sitting and roll down. See if you can slow it down and speed it up without compromising the quality. Rest on your back.

• Now imagine the movement as if you were on the roller. Can you design the movement in your imagination as if it was done perfectly? Effortlessly?

• Return to the roller. Repeat your original movement and see if it has changed in any way. If you still cannot do the movement without strain, return to the exploration process as a way to improve. Remember to check the other side for comparisons.

"Measure your mistakes and improvements." – Feldenkrais

XI **SWIMMER:** SU; this exercise is best done following the performance of the CAT/Camel Idea.
Lie on the roller with your head and hands resting on the floor. Your hands should be above your head and your legs should be stretched out long, away from your face.

• Think of your body drawn in five lines, with your middle line defined on the roller.

• Slowly slide your right hand away and lift your right arm off the floor. Notice your five lines. Avoid over-arching your low back and allow the back of your head to lift slightly from the floor. Lower your head and arm back down and repeat this five times, keeping your attention on your five lines.

• Now, lift your opposite leg (the left leg), again feeling the connections, and lower your leg back down. Repeat this exercise five times. Pause on the roller.

• Next, lift your left leg, right arm and head off the roller. Try and synchronize these parts as one unit. Feel where your counter pressure is. Repeat this step five times, then rest and slide off the roller and lie on your back, noticing any differences between the two sides.

• Return to the roller lying face down. Lift your left arm five times while you also slightly lift the back of your head. How does this side compare? Note where you press into the roller when you do this. Pause.

• Lift your opposite leg (the right leg), and repeat this movement five times. Pause.

• Combine your left arm, head and right leg, and synchronize them to lift at the same time. Distribute the effort evenly, avoiding any strain to your neck, back or anywhere else. Pause.

• Try lifting all four parts a little from the floor, allowing just a light touch with your fingers and toes on the floor. Balance in this position. Pause and lower back to the floor. Repeat this exercise five times.

• Roll gently off the roller and onto your back. Notice your back on the floor now. What is the impression you have of your back to the floor?

• Come back onto the roller, but this time on your back. Your knees are bent and your feet are on the floor. Gently rock back and forth to soften your back and then return to the floor. Compare the feeling of your back after performing these exercises and slowly stand up and walk around.

Can you set up 'idea like' conditions when you address other forms of strength training? Remember when you turn the brain on, more than your muscles are engaged.

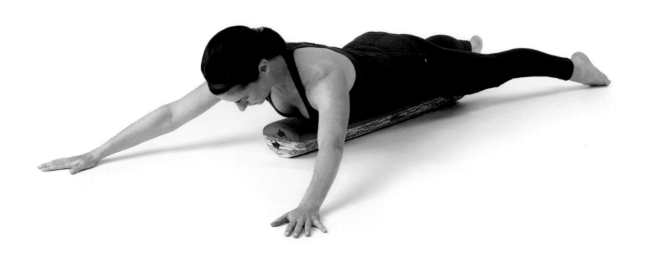

Besides varying the strength exercises by simply supplementing LINKS for the SMARTROLLER, here are some additional ideas to add to your exercises.

(I) PLANK: Place the LINKS, SD, and position your hands so your thumb is with your fingers—an ape hand. This position protects the joints of your thumb and wrists and supports your hand more anatomically.

- Position yourself like a cat on all fours with your knees directly under your hips. Roll up a mat to place under your knees if you have any trouble putting weight on them.

- Round and sag your spine, noting each segment of your back. Don't move so far as to stretch in this position. Make it an easy movement, making sure that you have full movement in your spine. Pause in the middle.

- Keeping your spine quiet and flat like a table, move only your shoulder blades away and towards your spine. Repeat this movement five to six times. Pause in the middle.

- Next, step your legs away from you, putting your weight onto your toes as if in a push up or plank position. Try and keep the shoulder blades quietly still, and flat on your back as you balance your weight evenly. Maintain this position for 60 seconds and then lower your knees to the floor.

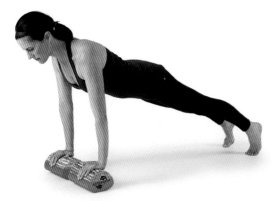

- Return to the plank position. As you maintain your alignment, lift your right leg and point your toes away from you. Lower your leg back to the floor and repeat this five times.

  Notice how your shoulders adapt to the movement. As you repeat this, observe how you stabilize yourself.

- Repeat this with your left leg. How does this side compare to the other side? Do this exercise slowly five times, then lower your knees down and gently round and sag your back a few times. Roll onto your back to finish and notice the feeling of your shoulder blades and spine on the floor.

(II) DIPS: Sit on the floor with your knees bent. Place the LINKS behind you and place one hand on each link.

- Anchor your feet into the floor. Press into your hands; straighten your elbows and lift your pelvis up off the floor. Pause and return your pelvis slowly to the floor.

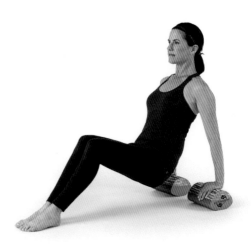

- Repeat this motion five times.

Variation: Sustain your pelvic lift and straighten and lift your right leg. Keeping your leg lifted, lower your pelvis back down. Lift your pelvis back up and return your right foot to the floor. Follow with your left foot and alternate your legs five times.

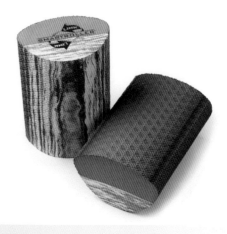

STANDING PELVIC HIKE: Stand near a wall with your right foot on one link and straighten your knee. With your left foot hanging off the ground and your left hip level with your right hip, slowly lower your left leg towards the floor. Do only the amount of movement that you can to keep your right knee straight.

• Repeat this movement five times.

• Step down off the link and walk around. Notice how your hips feel and compare.

• Repeat this for your right leg. Stand on the LINK with your left foot, straighten your left leg and lower your right hip down. How do they compare? Step onto the floor and notice the changes.

BUTTOCKS: Lie on the floor and place 2 LINKS under your pelvis. Prop up onto your forearms. Stabilize your position with your upper body and lift and lower your right leg a few inches off the floor. Feel the pressure under your pelvis on the two LINKS.

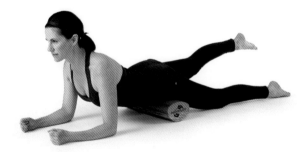

See if you can distribute your movement in such a way that you don't strain or collapse into your low back. Repeat this five times. Follow this exercise with your left leg. Slide the links out and roll onto your back. Scan your contact with the floor.

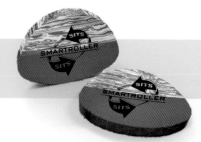

strength training
using your SITS

Exercise while you sit? Yes... you can.

Improve your strength through observing better alignment and reduce unwanted muscular resistance. Make skeletal awareness essential to your core workouts.

Props used are 1.5 lb. H$_2$O bottles, the BodyBlade®, resistance band, and Pilates ring. Choose one or more props depending on your time and interest. Grab your SMARTROLLER SITS, props and you are ready!

Sit in a stable chair without arm rests. Move to the edge of your chair. Place both feet flat on the floor. Notice how you are sitting. Compare the two sides of your body, noticing which sits bone you are sitting on. Observe how you are breathing. Are your shoulders level? Feel where your head is positioned. Does it tilt to the side? Is your head leaning forward or is it directly over your shoulders?

Remember to not make adjustments yet, only notice this before you start your SITS training and return to this scan afterward to see if you have adjusted to a better alignment through your exercise with awareness.

Place one SITS under each sit bone as described earlier and continue with the following exercises. Be sure to always start with the Body Resistance Only exercises (first three exercises) for preparation. The following exercises can be edited down to one prop or fewer repetitions, but take the time to feel the exercises with or without the SITS during and after the exercise.

(I) BODY RESISTANCE ONLY: These exercises will help you to find your best dynamic posture.

....

1. Slump and Lengthen: Did you know that your spine requires an auxiliary motion for reaching, bending and shock absorption? This is referred to as a kinematic chain, and it allows for the assembly of rigid parts (your bones) to be connected to create flexibility and motion. This piston-like action is for dynamic suspension in a healthy spine.

• Sitting at the edge of the chair, slowly shrink as if you are slumping. Allow your back to round and your shoulders to roll forward. Notice how you do this. See if you can shorten as opposed to leaning back. Be sure to move slowly. You should be able to count to five before you reach the end of the movement.

  How does the pressure change on your SITS? Take your time and feel all the parts of your back as you get lower.

• Next, press into the floor with both feet and lengthen your back as if you wanted to see over someone in front of you.

  As you do this slowly, feel how your spine gets longer through the direct pressure of your feet and SITS. See if you can visualize your whole spine as you do this. Can you picture this movement as if your spine acted like an accordion?

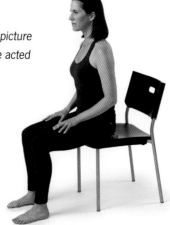

• Alternate these two movements and repeat this five times. Where have you see this before? Do you remember the action of the head and the pelvis when you did the pelvic clock? Pause in the middle.

Remove the SITS and repeat the slump and lengthening movements. Notice if you can feel your own sits bones more clearly now.

> **NOTE:** You begin by moving slowly with the easier motion of flexing or bending. This enables you to enlist more of your whole body into the action. Then, when you reverse the movement to extend up, you will be able to coordinate more of yourself into the movement.

2. Dips: This exercise will you help clarify the movements of your shoulders and your back muscles. Sit on a wide chair or bench. Place your hands in fists on your chair next to your hips. How much bend is in your elbows?

- While pressing your fists downward into the chair, slowly start to straighten your elbows. Do your shoulder blades move as you do this? In what direction? Repeat this five times.

  You should feel a slight lift of pressure under your SITS as you do this.

- Pause. Now, slowly shrink and shorten your body— as you did in the accordion movement from the last exercise—but let your elbows bend and straighten as you do this. Repeat this movement five times.

  Notice the relationship to your elbow bending and your trunk bending as you repeat this movement. Can you sense your shoulder blades moving?

- Now, push into your fists and straighten your elbows. Keep them in this position and, again, shrink and lengthen, but this time without bending in your elbows. Can you feel how one movement supports moving your shoulder blades and one does not?

- Remove the SITS. Is there a difference in your sitting height after doing this?

  See if you notice your shoulder blades and upper back muscles more clearly. Often, the chronic tensing of your shoulder blades can be what actually pulls your sitting posture downward.

3. Roll Down Forward: This is a good exercise for spinal coordination and articulation.

- Sit at the edge of the chair on your SITS, feet on the floor, and notice where your eyes are directed. Lengthen your spine as before and notice where you direct your eyes.

- Look in the direction of the horizon. Very slowly, start to look down.

  Does your head follow your movement? Only roll your eyes up and down a few times. Pause in the middle.

- Start with your eyes on the horizon and your weight balanced between your feet and on your SITS. Rest both hands on your thighs. Start to look down, and, as you roll your eyes downward, allow your spine to bend forward in sequential order. Think of bending over a large ball. Let your hands slide over your thighs and move towards your feet. Now, return back by pressing through both feet and SITS to reverse the movement. Stack your spine back up to the starting position, leaving your head for last. Notice how your eyes are involved with the movement. Can you sense when you breathe in and out? Be sure to only do only what is comfortable and easy. Repeat this five times.

- Remove your SITS and repeat the roll down exercise five times, noting where your points of contact with the floor and chair are located. This will help guide your skeletal awareness through your movement.

19 IDEA STRENGTH TRAINING USING YOUR SITS

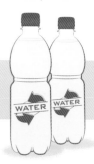

NOTE: The next exercises will use props for resistance. Your SITS are in place for five repetitions, then remove the SITS to repeat the same set for another five repetitions. This will provide a low-repetition circuit training at the same time as you improve your body awareness. If this is too much, explore removing the SITS at different times throughout the exercises to help you recognize your skeletal support.

H₂O BOTTLES OR FREE WEIGHTS: Here are some exercises that are easily done while sitting. If you don't have access to free weights, you can grab two large water bottles that usually equal about 1.5 pounds. Sit at the edge of the chair on your SITS, feet flat on the floor and hip-distance apart.

1. Diagonal A: With your right hand, take your one to two pound weight and reach your arm up overhead. Keep your elbow straight and have your right arm about a fist-space from your head. Your hand position is with your thumb directed behind you, as if you were hitch hiking. If you are doing this with a bottle, the bottle cap should point behind you.

- Begin by lowering your arm across your body diagonally, keeping your elbow straight. Rotate your arm in space to point your thumb downward, as if you are moving the weight in an orbital action. Move diagonally across your body to finish with the weight on your left thigh. The bottle cap will be pointed to your thigh.

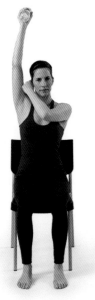
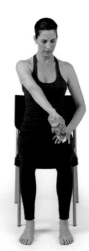

Once you understand the movement, can you feel the pressure shift under your SITS?

- Reverse the direction, rotating your right hand upward as you bring your arm back to your start position (bottle cap points behind you).

  Repeat this five times. Follow with the left arm and take note of any differences. Does one side seem more natural, smoother?

2. Diagonal B: With your right hand, hold the weight down at your side. Your palm will be facing backward with your thumb oriented toward your side.

- Start to lift the weight forwards across your body, towards your left ear. Allow your elbow to bend as you slowly rotate your arm to finish next to your left ear. Your thumb is now pointing forward. The bottle cap should be directed forward.

- Lower your arm slowly in the reverse direction in one smooth movement. The twisting movement is to be done continuously throughout the range, not all at once.

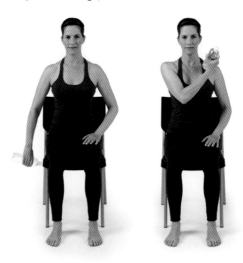

Once you understand the movement, can you feel the pressure shift slightly under your SITS? You want to sense this slight action while maintaining an even support and without adding unwanted tension in your body.

- Repeat this action five times.

- Follow with your left arm. How does this compare to your other arm?

3. Overhead Raise: Take both weights and raise them up towards your head. Your elbows should be bent, and your body should be balanced on your feet and both SITS.

• As you breathe in, lift both arms towards the sky, and then breathe out as you slowly lower them to your start position.

4. Chopping: Take both weights and raise them up over your head. Touch both weights together as if they are one. Your elbows will be straight.

• With your arms straight, bring them down towards your right knee as if you were chopping something and return back to your start position. Your spine will slightly bend but not collapse.

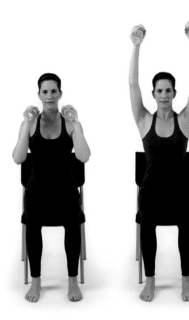

Once you understand the movement, can you feel the pressure under your SITS?

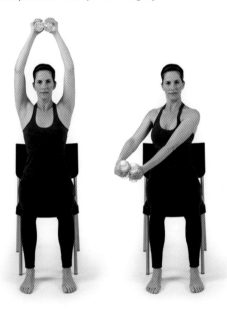

• Repeat this five times. Then repeat the movement with the opposite breath pattern. Which breath pattern seems more matched to the movement?

• Repeat this five times. Switch the chopping pattern to move towards your left knee. How do the two directions compare?

5. Seated Row: Take both weights and bring them in towards your chest with your elbows bent.

• As you straighten your arms directly out in front, you will simultaneously lean your body back, keeping your spine long but not rigid.

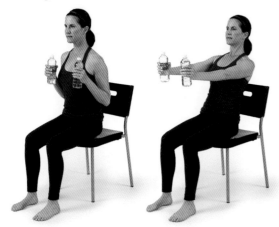

• Follow by reversing the movement and bending your elbows in towards your chest. Repeat this five times.

Once you understand the movement, can you feel the pressure change under your SITS?

6. Trunk Strengthening with Ribcage Arms: Take both weights and lift them to chest height with your elbows straight and arms directly in front.

• Keeping your spine long and feet in contact with the floor, lean backwards as you lift your arms directly up towards the sky. Pause, then lower your arms back out in front as you lean forward to your original position. Be aware that you should not shrug your shoulders towards your ears. Continue to breathe throughout the motion. Repeat this five times.

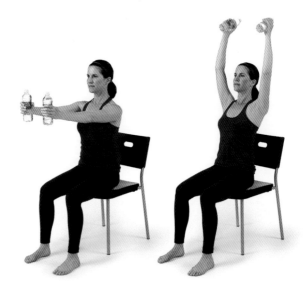

• See if you can connect to the muscles in the back of your thighs, as well as your deep abdominal contraction.

Once you have completed all six exercises from this set, remove the SITS, and repeat exercises one to six again. As you do the exercises, see if you can carry the image of the SITS and the balance of weight on your feet. If you continue, you can choose to use the SITS through some of the exercises and remove them as long as you remember to sense the space where the SITS were. This makes them effective sensory-motor learning tools.

III RESISTANCE BAND: For these exercises, you will anchor the resistance band as described in each exercise to create the necessary resistance. It is important to note that with all the exercises, there are two types of contraction. One is a contraction in your muscles with a movement made by shortening the angles of the body (concentric). When you reverse these angles of the body you are exercising the muscles by lengthening them (eccentrically). As mentioned earlier, research tells us that most of our sports and daily movements access more eccentric contractions. For the following set, be aware of the resistance you encounter when you return the band back to the resting position.

1. Hug a Tree: Sit at the edge of the chair on your SITS, feet on the floor, hip distance apart. Wrap the band behind your upper back near your shoulder blades and also around your hands and wrists to take out any slack. Your elbows will be slightly bent and out to the sides with your hands in front.

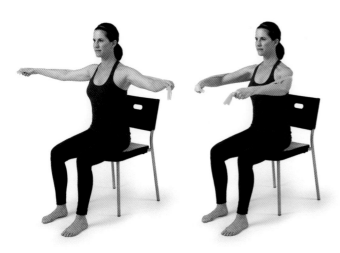

- Push your arms forward in a circular path as if you are hugging a tree to touch your hands together. Allow your spine to lengthen throughout the movement. Pause and then slowly return your hands back to the start position. Remember to resist the movement of the band so the action of the band does not do the movement for you (eccentric contraction).

   Repeat this movement five times. Breathe out when you move the arms inward and breathe in when you return them to their resting position.

2. Shoulder Wings (Serratus): Place the band in the same arrangement as it was in the Hug a Tree exercise. Extend your arms straight out in front.

- With your elbows straight, reach forward so your shoulder blades slide away from your spine. Pause. Then return to your start position. Make sure you keep your elbows straight. Try this without tensing your neck muscles or shrugging your shoulder blades upward.

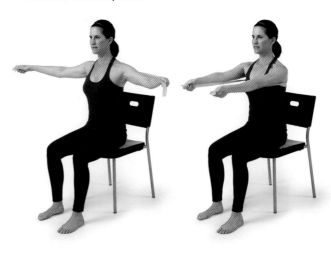

- Repeat this five times. Notice if your arms are different. By now, you are using and noting your differences to help improve your sensitivity to movement.

19 IDEA STRENGTH TRAINING USING YOUR SITS

3. Chest Expansion: Wrap the band around both hands in front of your body with your elbows bent to 90-degree angles and palms facing each other.

- Pull your hands apart against the resistance. As you do this, press gently into the floor and through your SITS to lengthen your spine. Pause.

- Slowly turn your head and look to your right, then to your left and back to the middle.

- Release the tension slowly and let your hands return to the starting position.

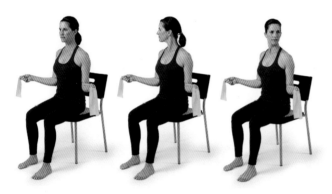

- Repeat the movement, but this time look to your left, then your right and back to the front. Continue the exercise five times as you alternate back and forth.

4. Frog Leg: Bend your right knee and slip the band around your right foot. Having your shoes on sometimes helps keep the band from slipping off your foot. Sit evenly on your SITS and your left foot. Do the next three exercises only with your right side and then repeat all three with your left side.

- Extend your right leg in the air. Resist the band and hold your foot a few inches from the floor. Pause. Return your leg back to the start position. Repeat this exercise five times.

5. Single Leg Bicycle: With the band wrapped around your right foot, extend your right foot out until your knee is straight with your leg lifted in the air.

- Bend your knee as if you were circling your foot around in a motion similar to pedaling a bicycle. Continue with the pedal motion five times.

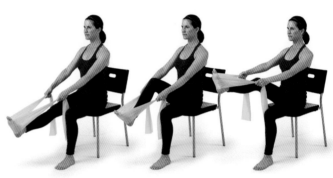

- Pause. Now reverse the circle five more times. Make the movement smooth and continuous. Rest your heel down for a moment before you continue on.

6. Single Leg Circles: Keep the band wrapped around your right foot and extend your right leg.

- With your right leg straight and a few inches from the floor, move your straight leg in a circle five times and then reverse the movement.

- Remove the band and notice the effect from using only one side. Now follow the last three exercises with the left leg.

- Remove the SITS. Feel your sitting posture. Walk around for a moment if you wish to continue.

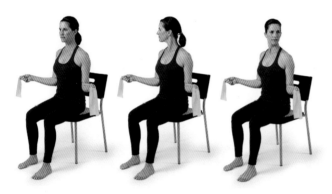

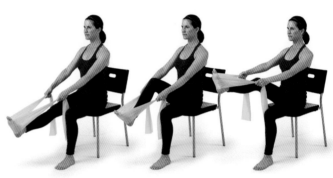

IV **PILATES RING:** If you do not have a Pilates ring, you can try these next exercises with a firm ball (approximately seven to eight inches.) Place the SITS under each sits bone.

1. Inner Thighs: Place the ring between your thighs just above your knees. Squeeze gently, pulse a few times while maintaining contact with your feet and SITS, and then release the contraction. Repeat this movement five times.

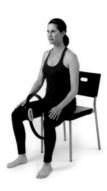

2. Abdominals and Triceps: Place the ring on top of your thighs. Push down on the ring with your extended arms and pulse down a few times. See if you can sense that you are getting taller as you do this. Maintaining your contacts, repeat this movement five times.

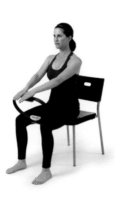

3. Inner Arms: With your arms out in front of you, place the ring in between your forearms. Squeeze the ring and pulse a few times with both arms. Notice how you engage your stomach muscles. Release the ring and squeeze again five times. Each time you squeeze the ring, see if you can get a little taller.

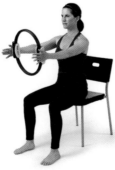

4. Mermaid: Place the ring in both hands overhead. Press gently down on both SITS and your heels, as you lengthen your spine. With only a slight squeeze with the ring, and without the pulses, slowly side-bend to the right. Take care to not collapse or lean over. Instead, imagine that there is an arch you are reaching over. Pause in this position and then return back to your start position. Repeat this movement five times. Then follow with the same steps on the left. Notice the differences.

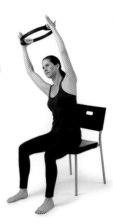

5. Back and Buttocks: Place the ring behind you, so it is against your middle back and the back of the chair. Press gently into the SITS and lengthen your spine. Keeping your spine long, press slowly into the ring. Feel what you use to do this. Pause and return to the start position. Repeat this movement five times.

Notice the engagement in your back, buttocks and thighs. If you are tensing elsewhere, direct your muscle recruitment to these prescribed areas.

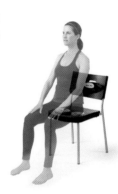

6. Trunk Twist: With your arms out in front of you, place the ring in between your forearms. Press into the SITS and into your feet. Maintain a light squeeze on the ring and slowly twist to the right. Maintain your length, pause and return to the middle. Repeat this movement to the right five times. Follow with turning to the left five times. Remove your SITS and notice your posture.

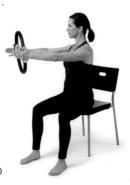

(V) BODYBLADE- With your weight balanced on your SITS and your feet on the floor, start these next exercises with the BodyBlade.

....

1. Chest Press with Abdominals:
With the BodyBlade in both hands and your spine kept long, tilt back from your hips and drive the BodyBlade forward and back in front of your body for 30 seconds. Continue the rhythmic forward and back motion as you hold this position. Feel the deep abdominal contraction while you hold your skeletal control. Return to sitting vertically and rest the BodyBlade on your lap.

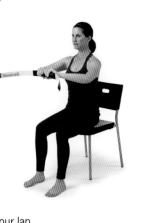

....

2. Obliques: Lift the BodyBlade up to shoulder height, oriented horizontally in a wide side position. Keeping your spine long, tilt back from your hips. Start driving the BodyBlade forward and back in front of you and slowly rotate to the right for 30 seconds. Continue driving the BodyBlade and hold this position. Maintaining the motion of

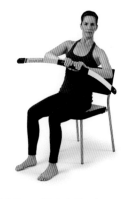

the BodyBlade, return to the middle and follow with twisting to the left for 30 seconds and hold. Remember to sense your SITS and weight through your heels. Once again, return to the middle, stop driving the BodyBlade and rest your arms on your lap.

....

3. Diagonals: Lift the BodyBlade with both hands horizontally in a wide side position overhead and slightly to the right, start driving (oscillating) the blade, and bring the BodyBlade diagonally down towards your left knee. Maintaining the motion of the blade, reverse the movement back up overhead. Observe what your eyes are doing. Can you direct the movement first with your eyes?

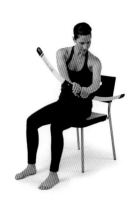

Repeat this five times and rest. Follow with the left side diagonal and compare the differences. As you take time to notice the differences, you may be able to access better choices to refine the exercises.

....

4. Single Punch: Place the BodyBlade in your right hand oriented vertically in a wide position as if you were going to punch forward and slightly to the right. Start driving the BodyBlade for 30 seconds while you slowly continue to move your arm more to the right. Return the BodyBlade to the middle and place it in your left hand. Continue with the BodyBlade oriented in the same vertical position as you direct it to the left for another 30 seconds. Go back and forth 5 times to each side. Rest as you need to.

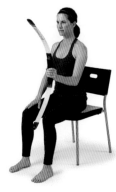

....

5. Rotator Cuff: Place the BodyBlade in your right hand, vertically oriented in front of your body in the wide side position, elbow bent to 90 degrees. Begin driving the blade forward and back and slowly rotate your arm internally and back to center, then externally and back to center. As a progression to this exercise, place the BodyBlade in your right hand, vertically oriented as before in front of your body. However, this time, position the blade in the narrow side position (looking at the thin side of the BodyBlade), elbows bent at 90 degrees, and begin driving the BodyBlade side to side. See if you can maintain this for 30 seconds and then try it with your left hand.

....

6. Overhead Pump: Take the BodyBlade in both hands, oriented vertically in front of your body in a wide side position, and lift it up overhead so the BodyBlade is now oriented horizontally parallel to the floor. Keeping your spine long, drive or oscillate the BodyBlade up and down for 30 seconds. As a progression to this exercise, in the same overhead position, orient the BodyBlade in the narrow side position and drive the BodyBlade left and right.

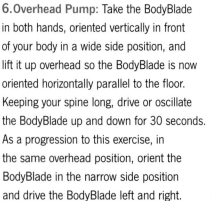
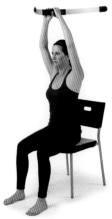

(VI) **ON TO THE FLOOR:** The next exercises are included at the end to accompany your sitting program on the floor. The essence of the exercises completed with your SITS will help accommodate the long sitting positions required by these familiar Pilates and Yoga routines. You may add props as an option.

1. Spine Stretch: Sit on the floor and slide your SITS under each of your sits bones. Lengthen and spread your legs apart. Place your hands on the floor in between your legs and slide your hands forward. Curl your spine and draw your belly in. Go as far as you can comfortably move and then return to your start position. Repeat this movement five times. Remove your SITS and rest.

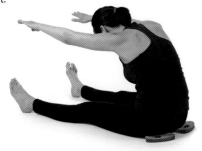

Note: Although it is common practice to draw the belly in, this is not recommended to be done as a habit at all times. The benefit here is to practice the feeling of the contraction as well as when you disengage the abdominals. That way you aren't chronically holding these muscles so they are available for lengthening.

2. The Saw: Sit on the floor as shown; slide a SITS under each sits bone. Lengthen and spread your legs apart. Bring your arms up and out to the sides (shoulder-high). Twist from your trunk only to the right. Bend forward and downward until your left hand crosses and rests diagonally on your right foot. Slide your left hand in a saw-like motion three times. Return back to sitting up and return to the middle. Twist your body to the left. Bend forward and downward until your right hand crosses your left foot. Slide your right hand forward in a saw-like motion three times. Return back up to sitting and twist back to the middle. Repeat this five times to each side. Remove your SITS and rest.

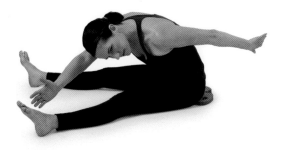

3. The Spine Twist: Sit on the floor as shown, legs together, and slide a SITS under each sits bone. Bring your arms out to the side, shoulder-width, palms down. Twist your head and body to the right as you balance your weight on your SITS. Pause and then turn to the middle. Twist your body to the left, again, balancing your weight on your SITS and then returning to the middle. Repeat the movement in each direction five times. Remove your SITS and rest.

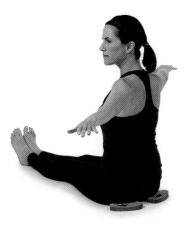

Now that you have used props to improve your body awareness, try these ideas to find more optimal ways to transition your everyday movements.

To stand upright, "*Take a Bow*": This will help you find a better standing support that reduces a protruding abdomen – a shrinking posture – while you reduce strain on your spine. This cue will help you include your hips in your standing balance.

To start, notice how your weight is distributed under your feet. Can you sense how tall you are just by feeling? Are you bent forward, backward or straight over your hip joints? Next, look from side to side and see how far you go. Notice how you do this. Pick a point in the distance to refer back to as a measure of how far you turn.

Now, take a bow by hinging at your hips and allowing your spine to move as a unit. Do this several times to help you notice the bend in your hips. Repeat this several times, each time reducing your movement. As you make the movement smaller and smaller, draw more attention to the details. When do you breathe in and out? Does the pressure change under your feet? Do your toes remain relaxed?

After you have completed this exercise, pause where you feel that your upright position is vertical, or plumb. This is a dynamic reference, not a place to park. To avoid getting fixed in this position, turn and look around yourself. Can you look farther to the side? Try this: shift your hips forward and turn to look around. Notice that you will turn less and are unable to access your legs with the turn.

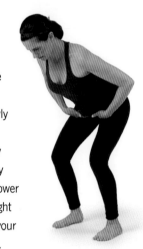

To bend down, "*Bow and Buckle*": This idiom is used to help elicit a new way for you to bend and lift with the best body mechanics. Remember the hinge movement you just did for standing? Start to slowly hinge from your hips. Now, buckle or bend your knees as you continue to bend—"bow and buckle." You will see that you are lowering your center of gravity with your whole body. To rise, reverse and combine both movements with smooth synchronization. Try to do this slowly and carefully, so that you allow yourself time to feel how your body does this. Think of leap frog. It may help you to understand how your lower body is designed to bring your weight upward. This helps you distribute your body's mechanics more effectively.

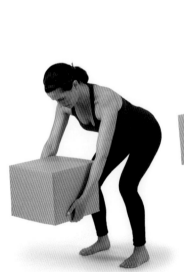
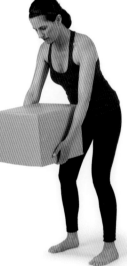

Often we are told to lift objects with our legs, but the problem with this is the tendency to only bend from our knees without the integration of our hips. Remember, your hips are the largest joints and should be used for large tasks.

"There is a distinct advantage of reversibility: Not only does the movement become more fluid, but it also has a greater range of adaptability." – Elizabeth Beringer

To sit down,
"Squat to Sit":

In our society, we are less accustomed to sitting down by squatting. However, if you start to sit as if you wanted to squat to the floor, you will find it easier on all your joints. Find your chair, follow the bow and buckle approach to bending and lower yourself slowly down into the chair. Practice the act of completing only part of the movement and return to standing. Can you do this without interfering with your breathing? Where do you direct your eyes? If you had to suddenly stop the movement, could you? Notice your body when you approach the last few inches from the chair. Over time, this will allow you to strengthen your hips and buttock muscles. These muscles are some of your most sustainable muscles for dynamic stability.

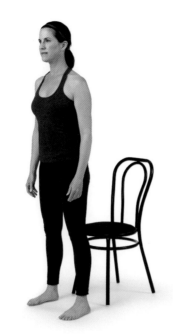

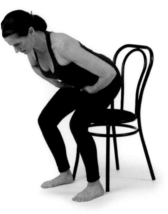

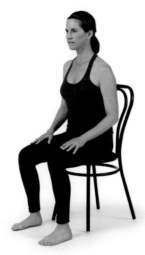

To stand up, find *"Reversibility/Sit to Stand":*
When you rise from sitting, first think about the way you sat in the bow and buckle approach. Can you think about reversing this action, using the same easy approach to stand up? Optimal movement is easily reversible. You will see this when you watch athletes, such as golfers or martial artists, who are able to fine-tune their skill with such clarity that they can stop and reverse their movement at any time.

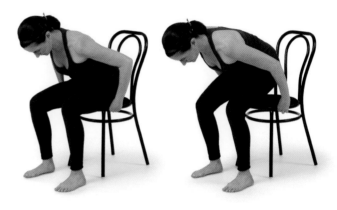

Come to the edge of your chair, and feel where you place your feet. Notice the bones under your bottom, your sits bones, and hinge forward until you start to feel yourself begin to lift the pressure off your sits bones. This is usually far more forward than you are used to, but start to practice rising from a sit position in this way. Once your weight is transferred forward like this, notice how the back of your neck feels.

Can you allow your head to hang loosely down until you start to rise to stand? Just by changing what muscles you use to stand with, you will have better overall balance and less joint strain. Practice this every time you rise from a chair to promote your vitality!

As a physical therapist, I am accustomed to setting up programs to support diligence in improving daily habits of practice. I only do this after there is an established practice and understanding of awareness. This way, the student/patient is already practicing how they attend to their movement. I have selected a few profiles that may clarify ideas in action. The following templates were designed to show how SMART ideas can be used for certain styles of training.

- Suggested schedule: Four week program, 15 to 20 minutes per idea with a new idea every other day.

- Once all the selected sequences are completed, a ten minute touch-up with a suggested brief review of each idea is to be completed within four weeks.

- This alternative approach to training will help maintain and support ways to erase poor habits and help support efficacy with basic dynamic skills such as better posture, balance, core training and coordination.

....

Teenage Texter/Soccer Player: Posture is one of the many battles parents have with teenagers. Heavy backpacks, large growth spurts and reduced outdoor play are all part of the cause. Adding to this problem is the limited use of their eyes. Eyes are extremely important in movement and, when you look at smaller spaces, there is added body tension.

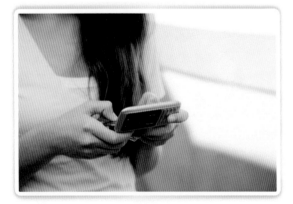

The limited success in changing or correcting postural habits is partly due to the way good dynamic posture is taught. In the absence of outdoor play in nature, these Smart Ideas are designed to support the natural use of children's own developmental tools that will encourage a better and more

dynamic posture. Set aside time for your teen to complete the ideas with some negotiations to make it more like a game and less like homework. You can read the puzzles out loud or record them ahead of time and have your teen listen to them on their own. Here are the suggested choices to help create better posture and to support new movement learning and their sports training.

Weekend Warrior/Golfer: Many people discover after an injury or two, they no longer can work at a desk during the workweek and run out to play on the weekend without consequences. Despite hitting the gym after work, there is less full body activity throughout the day. Many movements that were inherently available become

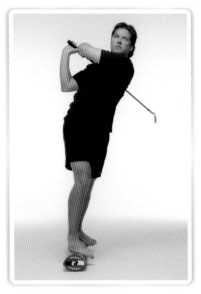

forgotten. With these SR ideas, more movement choices can be available and ready for use.

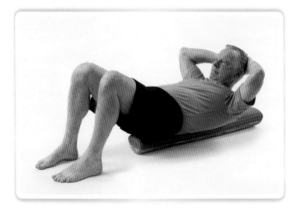

Senior Writer/Balance Challenges: Because sitting is a way of life for writers, the issues of poor balance may arise even earlier. Balance and improved posture can be improved easily with regular use of the SMARTROLLER.

"What you truly learn best will appear
to you later as your own discovery." – Moshe Feldenkrais

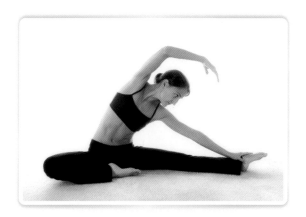

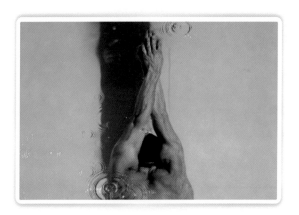

Pilates Instructor: In my experience, good Pilates instructors are self learners and what they learn for themselves is often the inspiration for what they teach to their clients. All of the movement sequences are appropriate for this person.

Triathlete: Triathletes have many training needs. Even though they are committed to train to exceed the limits, they are not exempt from what they can learn. By using sensory motor tools, they may develop better skeletal support to free their muscles for action. Here are some ideas for whole body training, economical athletic stance on a bicycle and finding balance and propulsion in the water.

RECOMMENDED ESSENTIAL IDEAS

IDEA	1	2	3	4	5	6	7	8	9	10	11	12	13	14	15	16	17	18	19
Texter		●		●	●	●	●		●		●	●	●		●	●	●		
Warrior		●	●	●	●	●	●	●	●			●	●	●	●	●			
Senior	●	●	●	●	●	●	●		●			●		●		●			●
Pilates	●	●	●	●	●			●	●		●	●		●			●		●
Swim	●	●	●	●	●			●	●	●	●					●	●		
Run	●	●		●		●	●	●			●	●		●	●	●	●		
Cycle	●		●	●				●	●		●		●	●	●		●	●	●

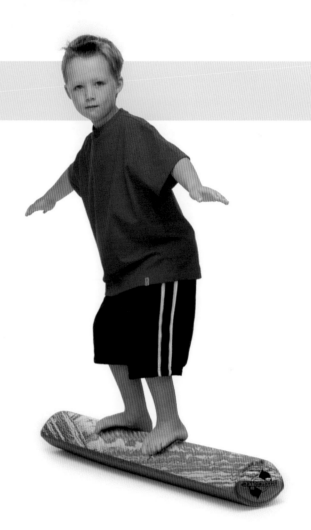

conclusion

Hopefully, you have gained some new ideas to improve your movement IQ. Remember to be patient with yourself when learning something new. Consider making your everyday movements a novel and refreshing way to explore the use of gravity with an improved sensitivity to movement.

This project is a work in progress, a first approximation. I would like to hear your ideas, experiences and suggestions.

Remember to create a Smart Way to move with renewable strength and vitality.

— Stacy Barrows, PT, GCFP, PMA Pilates teacher

acknowledgements

I am indebted to Dr. Moshe Feldenkrais for helping me become a better learner and to my wonderful trainers, the late Mark Reese, Ralph Strauch and many others who helped me access Feldenkrais' mission to help people tap into their own capacity to improve. I could not have made it this far without the help and guidance of many colleagues, friends and family. I extend my sincere gratitude to my fellow physical therapists, Feldenkrais practitioners and Pilates Instructors. A special thank you to Sara Dacklin for her highly professional photos and also for her guidance to help me transform with Pilates concepts.

This process has taken a considerable amount of time, and it has allowed me to learn from many of my students and patients. Without them, my own practical learning focused on teaching others would not be possible. And a very generous thank you to the many contributing editors of these pages, specifically Matt Barrows, Michael Sigman, Pat Haney, Marci Spiegler, Edward Yu, Cathy Lindvall, Karen Klingel, Shari Schroeder, Bruce Hymanson, Ellen Solloway, Carey Haskell, Elizabeth Davidow, Paula Batson, Marie José Blom, and the list goes on....

Thank you to my parents who encouraged me to follow my passions. Daniel and Scott Barrows, from the bottom of my heart, thank you for your reassurance and inspiration.

Thank you, Matt Barrows. You are my true compass in life. There are not enough words to express how much I want to thank you for your unconditional love and support, which has always been present since we met years ago.

references and suggested reading list

NEUROPLASTICITY

Bolte-Taylor, J. MY STROKE OF INSIGHT: Penguin Group Inc., New York, NY; 2006.

Brown, Stuart. PLAY: HOW IT SHAPES THE BRAIN, OPENS THE IMAGINATION, AND INVIGORATES THE SOUL: New York; 2009.

Begley, S. TRAIN YOUR MIND, CHANGE YOUR BRAIN: Ballantine Books, New York; 2007.

Blakeslee, S. & M. THE BODY HAS A MIND OF ITS OWN: Random House, Inc. New York; 2007.

Doidge, N. THE BRAIN THAT CHANGES ITSELF: Penguin Group Inc., New York, NY; 2007. <www.optp.com>

Howard, P. THE OWNER'S MANUAL TO THE BRAIN, EVERYDAY APPLICATIONS FROM MIND-BRAIN RESEARCH: Bard Press, Austin, TX; 2006.

Reilly, M. PLAY AS EXPLORATORY LEARNING: Sage Publications, Beverly Hills/London; 1974.

Schwartz, J. & S. Begley. THE MIND AND THE BRAIN: Regan Books, Harper Collins Publishers; 2002.

Siegel, D. MINDSIGHT: Bantam Books, New York; 2010.

SCIENTIFIC AND EDUCATIONAL SUPPORT FOR THE FELDENKRAIS METHOD

Allen, C. & C. Montgomery. GAIT AS AN ASSESSMENT AND INTERVENTION TOOL: A CASE STUDY: www.ilcma.com; 2007.

Alon, R. MINDFUL SPONTANEITY: LESSONS IN THE FELDENKRAIS METHOD: North Atlantic Books, Berkeley, California; 1996.

Barrows, S. THE FUTURE OF RESEARCH IN THE FELDENKRAIS METHOD: <http://www.iffresearchjournal.org/1barrows2007.htm>

Beringer, E. EMBODIED WISDOM: North Atlantic Books, Berkeley, CA; 2010 <www.optp.com>

Bersin, D, M. Reese. RELAXERCISE: Harper Collins, New York, NY; 1990.

Brown, G. A MANUAL THERAPIST GUIDE TO MOVEMENT: Churchill Livingstone, Elsevier, Edinburgh; 2006.

Burgess, R. A GUIDE TO BODY SENSE: Skeletal Life Publishers, Woleboro, NH; 2008.

Connors, K., M. Galea & C. Said. AN INVESTIGATION INTO FELDENKRAIS MOVEMENT CLASSES AND THEIR EFFECT ON BALANCE IN OLDER ADULTS: Melbourne University; 2007.

Doidge, N. NEW HOPE FOR ACHING, CREAKY YUPPIE BODIES: National Post, 1999; copyright Norman Doidge 2009 <http://www.feldenkraiscentre.com/pdfs/Doidge%20article.pdf>

Dean, J. & S. Barrows. THE EFFECT OF THE FELDENKRAIS METHOD AWARENESS THROUGH MOVEMENT WITH PEOPLE WITH FIBROMYALGIA: IFF Research Journal; 2007. <http://feldenkrais-method.org/en/search/node/dean>

Extensive research library/ PubMed search: <http://www.ncbi.nlm.nih.gov/pubmed?Db=pubmed&term=feldenkrais> and <http://feldenkrais-method.org/en/node/205>

Feldenkrais, M. AWARENESS THROUGH MOVEMENT: New York, N Y, Harper and Row; 1972.

Feldenkrais, M. HIGHER JUDO: North Atlantic Books, Berkeley, CA 2010; Original 1952.

Feldenkrais, M. POTENT SELF: North Atlantic Books, Berkeley, CA; 1985.

Heggie, J. SOME THOUGHTS ON THE RELATIONSHIP BETWEEN: VISION, PROPRIOCEPTION AND KINESTHETICS: Journal of Behavioral Optometry, Vol. 4/1993/Number 4/page 95-97.

Ofir, R. THE FELDENKRAIS METHOD: ON THE IMPORTANCE AND POTENCY OF SMALL AND SLOW MOVEMENTS; PT Forum; 9 (42):1-5. 1990.

Stephens J., Davidson J., DeRosa J., Kriz M., Saltzman, N. LENGTHENING THE HAMSTRING MUSCLES WITHOUT STRETCHING USING AWARENESS THROUGH MOVEMENT: Phys Ther 86: 1641-1650; 2006.

Thelan, E. MOTOR DEVELOPMENT: A NEW SYNTHESIS: American Psychologist, 79-95: Feb; 1995.

Weil, A. THE FELDENKRAIS METHOD, MOVING WITH EASE: SELF HEALING, May 1998. <http://www.feldenkraiscentre.com/pdfs/Weil%20article2.pdf>

FELDENKRAIS SUPPORTING PERFORMANCE

Barrows, S. YOU'RE ON A ROLL...ER: Golf for Women; 140-144; March/April 1997.

Heggie, J. RUNNING WITH THE WHOLE BODY: North Atlantic Books, Berkley, CA; 1996.

Heggie, J. SKIING WITH THE WHOLE BODY: North Atlantic Books, Berkley, CA; 1993.

Higgins, A. BODY OF KNOWLEDGE: Massachusetts, <www.kinestheticedge.com>; 2007.

Higgins, A. KINESTHETIC EDGE FOR GOLFERS: Massachusetts, <www.kinestheticedge.com>

Kimn, P. WALKING, NATURE'S PERFECT EXERCISE: Painfreechoices, Evanston, Il; 2008 <www.optp.com>

McIntyre, M. UNLOCK THE TRUNK: Skiing; 139-144; October 1992.

Parker, I. BEYOND CONVENTIONAL EXERCISE: Audio tape, Feldenkrais Conference; 1995.

Yu, E. THE ART OF SLOWING DOWN: A SENSE-ABLE APPROACH TO RUNNING: Panenthea Books, Harrisburg, PA; 2010.

ANATOMY, IMAGERY AND MOVEMENT

Baniel, A. MOVE INTO LIFE: Harmony Books, NY, 2009

Barrows, S. ROLLER REHAB: EXERCISES USING FOAM ROLLERS: Physical Therapy Products; 44-47, May-June, 2002.

Berthoz, A. THE BRAIN'S SENSE OF MOVEMENT: Harvard University Press, Cambridge, MA; 2000.

Cook, G. MOVEMENT: FUNCTIONAL MOVEMENT SYSTEMS SCREENING: On Target Publications, Santa Cruz, 2010.

Corning-Creager, C. THERAPEUTIC EXERCISE USING THE FOAM ROLLER: 1996. <www.oplp.com>

Dowd, I. TAKING ROOT TO FLY: Articles on Functional Anatomy, Irene Dowd, 1995.

Franklin, E. DYNAMIC IMAGERY: Human Kinetics, Champaign, Il, 1996. <www.optp.com>

Galante, L. TAI CHI: THE SUPREME ULTIMATE: Samuel Weiser, Inc., York Beach, ME; 1981.

Knott, M. & D. Voss. PROPRIOCEPTIVE NEUROMUSCULAR FACILITATION: Harper and Row, Hagerston, MD; 1968.

Meeks, S. WALK TALL: Triad Publishing Co. Gainsville, FA; 2010. <www.optp.com>

Myers, T. ANATOMY TRAINS: Elsevier, Edinburgh, London, 2009. <www.optp.com>

Pilates, J. RETURN TO LIFE: Pilates Method Alliance, Inc. Fl. 2003, 2005. (original ©Joseph H. Pilates 1945)

Quebedeux, B. POSTURE WITH A PURPOSE: audio-recording, 2010. <www.optp.com>

Reese, M. Notes and Transcripts of the Los Angeles Feldenkrais Professional Training; 1994.

Rywerant, Y. ACQUIRING THE PROFESSION: Tel Aviv, Israel, 2000.

Rywerant, Y. THE FELDENKRAIS METHOD: TEACHING BY HANDLING: Keats Publishing, Inc. New Canaan, Connecticut, 1983.

Sahrmann, S. DIAGNOSIS AND TREATMENT OF MOVEMENT IMPAIRMENT SYNDROMES: Minneapolis, MN, 2005. <www.optp.com>

Shafarman, S. AWARENESS HEALS: THE FELDENKRAIS METHOD FOR DYNAMIC HEALTH: Da Capo, Cambridge, MA, 1997.

Swartzlander, B. OUTSIDE THE BOX: Advance for Physical Therapists & Physical Therapy Assistants; August, 2008.

Sweigard, L. HUMAN MOVEMENT POTENTIAL, ITS IDEOKINETIC FACILITATION: Dodd, Mead, NEW YORK, NY; 1978.

Schmidt, R. MOTOR LEARNING AND PERFORMANCE: Human Kinetics, Champagne, Il: 2000, 2004, 2008.

Schultz, L.& R. Feitis. THE ENDLESS WEB: FASCIAL ANATOMY AND PHYSICAL REALITY: Berkeley, CA: North Atlantic Books; 1996.

Strauch, R. LOW STRESS COMPUTING: USING AWARENESS TO AVOID RSI, A FELDENKRAIS APPROACH: Pacific Palisades, CA, 1997.

Strauch, R. THE REALITY ILLUSION: SOMATIC OPTIONS: Pacific Palisades, CA, 2000.

Todd, M. THE THINKING BODY: Princeton Book Company, Hightstown, NJ, 1937.

Vleming, Mooney, Dorman, Snijders, Stoeckart. MOVEMENT, STABILITY & LOW BACK PAIN: Churchill Livingstone, New York, 1997.

Wildman, F. BUSY PERSON'S GUIDE TO EASIER MOVEMENT: Intelligent Body Press, Berkeley, CA; 2006.

Wildman, F. CHANGE YOUR AGE: Da Capo Books, Philadelphia, PA; 2010.

7th Interdisciplinary World Congress on Low Back Pain, BALANCED SOLUTIONS: EFFECTIVE IMPLEMENTATION OF EVIDENCE BASED RESEARCH: Los Angeles, CA; 2010.

GENERAL

Doyle, A. THE ORIGINAL ILLUSTRATED SHERLOCK HOLMES: New Jersey.
Edmonson, A. A FULLER EXPLANATION: THE SYNERGETIC GEOMETRY OF R. BUCKMINSTER FULLER: Emergent World Press, Pueblo, CO; 2007.
Goleman, D. EMOTIONAL INTELLIGENCE: Bantam Books, New York, NY; 1997.

ADDITIONAL RESOURCES, LINKS AND BLOGS

To avoid tedious typing of url links, go to *www.SMARTROLLER.net* for listings.

Alon, R. Bones for Life: <www.bonesforlife.com>; Movement Nature Meant: <http://www.youtube.com/watch?v=igpJeOkgfzw>
Barrows, S. Century City Physical Therapy, Inc.: <http://www.centurycitypt.com>
Barrows, S. Roll up to sit: <http://www.youtube.com/watch?v=LjIjGY0SymY>
Burgess, R. The Feldenkrais Method: <http://www.efeld.com/>
Campbell, V. Brain Science podcast: <http://www.brainsciencepodcast.com/>
Dellman, R. Embodied Life: <http://www.russelldelman.com/>
Hargrove, T. <http://toddhargrove.wordpress.com/>
Harris, M. Feldenkrais Centre: <http://www.feldenkraiscentre.com/>
Feldenkrais Center of Houston: <http://houstonfeldenkrais.com/>
Feldenkrais Guild: <www.feldenkrais.com>
Feldenkrais at Home: <http://feldenkraisathome.com/w/>
Feldenkrais Institute: <http://www.feldenkraisinstitute.com/>
Feldenkrais Movement Institute: <http://www.feldenkraisinstitute.org/>
Feldenkrais, the next 25 years: <http://www.thenext25years.com/>
Feldenkrais Resources: <http://www.feldenkraisresources.com/>
Feldenkrais Way: <http://feldenkraisway.com/>
Feldscinet.org. <http://www.feldscinet.org/>
Goldfarb, L. Mind in Motion: <http://www.mindinmotion-online.com/>
Heffernan, A: <http://www.malepatternfitness.com/; Experience Life magazine "Feldenkrais Fix", November, 2009.
Heartmath: <www.heartmath.org>
Haller, J. Inside Moves: < http://www.insidemoves.org/>
Jose, M: <http://pilatesinspiration.com/>
Laughlin, T. Total Immersion swimming: <http://www.totalimmersion.net/>
Nielsen, M. <http://www.top-form-fitness.com/articles/No-Foam-Roller.pdf>
Open ATM: <http://openatm.org/>
Leri, D: <http://www.semiophysics.com/>
Posit Science: <http://merzenich.positscience.com/>
Questal, A. Uncommon Sensing: <http://www.uncommonsensing.com/-FELDENKRAIS-R-PROFESSIONAL-.html>
Rolf, Ida: <http://www.rolfguild.org/>
Soloway, E: <soloway-feldenkrais.com>
SomaSimple: <http://www.somasimple.com/>
Scleip, R: <http://www.somatics.de/>
Spiegler, M: <http://www.altmd.com/Specialists/Marci-Spiegler>
Strauch, R: < http://www.somatic.com/>
Weiner, M: <http://martinweiner.com/>

index

Awareness Through Movement®: "The Feldenkrais Method® is expressed in two parallel forms: Awareness Through Movement® and Functional Integration®. Awareness Through Movement consists of verbally directed movement sequences presented primarily to groups. There are several hundred hours of Awareness Through Movement lessons. A lesson generally lasts from thirty to sixty minutes. Each lesson is usually organized around a particular function. In Awareness Through Movement lessons, people engage in precisely structured movement explorations that involve thinking, sensing, moving, and imagining. Many are based on developmental movements and ordinary functional activities. Some are based on more abstract explorations of joint, muscle, and postural relationships. The lessons consist of comfortable, easy movements that gradually evolve into movements of greater range and complexity. There are hundreds of Awareness Through Movement lessons contained in the Feldenkrais Method that vary, for all levels of movement ability, from simple in structure and physical demand to more difficult lessons." <www.feldenkrais.com>

Body Image: According to Paul Schilder, body image "refers to the mental pictures we have of our bodies or the way our bodies appear to us. The body image stems from learned attitudes about your body." [1]

Body schema: "...is a physiological construct. Your brain creates it from the interaction of touch, vision, proprioception, balance, and hearing. ...Your body schema is also informed by a library of what people call 'muscle memories', although the term is rather inaccurate. These memories actually reside in the brain's motor maps, not down in the muscles proper, as the term suggests. The body schema is a felt sense based on physical properties of your body." [2]

Buckminster Fuller: "R. Buckminster Fuller was a renowned 20th century inventor and visionary born in Milton, Massachusetts on July 12, 1895. Dedicating his life to making the world work for all of humanity, Fuller operated as a practical philosopher who demonstrated his ideas as inventions that he called "artifacts." Fuller did not limit himself to one field but worked as a 'comprehensive anticipatory design scientist' to solve global problems surrounding housing, shelter, transportation, education, energy, ecological destruction, and poverty. Throughout the course of his life Fuller held 28 patents, authored 28 books, received 47 honorary degrees. And while his most well known artifact, the geodesic dome, has been produced over 300,000 times worldwide, Fuller's true impact on the world today can be found in his continued influence upon generations of designers, architects, scientists and artists working to create a more sustainable planet." <http://bfi.org/>

Fascia: is a type of connecting tissue that surrounds muscles, groups of muscles, blood vessels, organs and nerves and joins together these structures throughout the body. This tissue is supplied with nerves that are assumed to serve a proprioceptive and pain receiving function. This tissue acts as a bodywide interconnecting network and is considered our largest sensory organ. Forces that transmit through the fascia are important in the understanding of human biomechanics. Recent studies show that fascial tissues are commonly used for dynamic energy storage for such activities as jumping and or running.

Feldenkrais Method®: "The Feldenkrais Method is named after its originator, Dr. Moshe Feldenkrais, D.Sc. (1904-1984), a Russian born physicist, judo expert, mechanical engineer and educator. The Feldenkrais Method is a form of somatic education that uses gentle movement and directed attention to improve movement and enhance human functioning. Through this Method, you can increase your ease and range of motion, improve your flexibility and coordination, and rediscover your innate capacity for graceful, efficient movement. These improvements will often generalize to enhance functioning in other aspects of your life." <www.feldenkrais.com>

[1,2] Blakeslee, S. and M. Blakeslee: THE BODY HAS A MIND OF ITS OWN

Feldenkrais Practitioner: "All Feldenkrais practitioners must complete 740-800 hours of training over a 3 to 4 year period. Trainees participate in Awareness Through Movement and Functional Integration lessons, lectures, discussions, group process and videos of Dr. Feldenkrais teaching. Eventually students teach Awareness Through Movement and Functional Integration under supervision. Trainees gradually acquire knowledge of how movement and function are formed and organized. This extensive subjective experience forms the basis from which she/he will learn to work with others. The main purpose of the training is for the trainees to acquire for themselves a deep understanding of movement and its formation, to become aware of their own movement, to become astute observers of movement in others, and to be able to teach other people to enlarge their awareness and movement skills. The training process is based upon the vast body of knowledge Dr. Feldenkrais introduced. Since he integrated into his body of learning theory aspects from a variety of scientific fields such as Newtonian mechanics, physics, neurophysiology, movement development, biology and learning theories, some of these aspects are presented in the training program for the trainee to comprehend the theoretical background of the method." <www.feldenkrais.com>

Flow: Mihaly Csikszentmihalyi defined flow as "being completely involved in an activity for its own sake. The ego falls away. Time flies. Every action, movement, and thought follows inevitably from the previous one, like playing jazz. Your whole being is involved, and you're using your skills to the utmost."[3] Csikszentmihalyi was one of the founders of positive psychology.

Functional Integration®: "Functional Integration is another form of expressing the Feldenkrais Method. Just as Feldenkrais practitioners can guide people through movement sequences verbally in Awareness Through Movement®, they also guide people through movement with gentle, non-invasive touching in Functional Integration. Functional Integration is a hands-on form of tactile, kinesthetic communication. The Feldenkrais practitioner communicates to the student how he/she organizes his/her body and hints, through gentle touching and movement, how to move in more expanded functional motor patterns. The Functional Integration lesson should relate to a desire, intention, or need of the student. The learning process is carried out without the use of any invasive or forceful procedure. Through rapport and respect for the student's abilities, qualities, and integrity, the practitioner/teacher creates an environment in which the student can learn comfortably." <www.feldenkrais.com>

Iliotibial band: is a fibrous thickening of the tensor fasciae latae, which extends from the iliac crest to the lateral condyle of the tibia along the outside of the thigh.

Neuroplasticity: "Refers to the ability of neurons to forge new connections, to blaze new paths through the cortex, even to assume new roles. In shorthand, neuroplasticity means rewiring the brain."[4]

Pilates Method Alliance®: "Founded in 2001, the Pilates Method Alliance is the professional association and certifying agency for Pilates teachers. For the past decade, Pilates teachers from around the world have worked together to create a unified community, to share knowledge and information, and, most importantly, to establish the practice of teaching Pilates as a profession. To that end, in 2005 the PMA launched the only third-party professional certification exam in the Pilates industry." <www.pilatesmethodalliance.org>

---

[3] Csikszentmihalyi, M. FLOW: THE PSYCHOLOGY OF OPTIMAL EXPERIENCE
[4] Schwartz, J. & S. Begley: THE MIND AND THE BRAIN

Proprioception: the neuromuscular system's internal feedback mechanism that tells you where you are in space and the relation of your body parts to the whole.

Ramachandran, V.S.: "V.S. Ramachandran is Director of the Center for Brain and Cognition and Professor with the Psychology Department and Neurosciences Program at the University of California, San Diego, and Adjunct Professor of Biology at the Salk Institute. Ramachandran initially trained as a doctor and subsequently obtained a Ph.D. from Trinity College at the University of Cambridge. Ramachandran's early work was on visual perception but he is best known for his experiments in behavioral neurology which, despite their apparent simplicity, have had a profound impact on the way we think about the brain. He has been called 'the Marco Polo of neuroscience' by Richard Dawkins and 'the modern Paul Broca' by Eric Kandel." <http://cbc.ucsd.edu/ramabio.html>

Rolf, Ida: "Ida P. Rolf, a native New Yorker, graduated from Barnard College in 1916; in 1920 she earned a Ph.D. in biological chemistry from the College of Physicians and Surgeons of Columbia University. She was committed to the scientific point of view, and yet many breakthroughs came intuitively through the work she did with chronically disabled persons unable to find help elsewhere. This was the work eventually to be known as Structural Integration." <www.rolfguild.org>

Rotator cuff: The rotator cuff muscles are four muscles and their tendons that are attached to the shoulder joint and function as a dynamic stabilizer and support for shoulder mechanics.

Soft tissue: tissue that connects, supports, or surrounds other structures and organs (e.g., tendons, ligaments, fascia, epithelium, fat, muscles, nerves and blood vessels).

Todd, Mabel: author of *The Thinking Body* (1972) and major contributor the concept of ideokinesis, overlapping the work of Heinrich Kosnick and Lulu Sweigard. Mabel Todd taught at Columbia University Teacher's College and experienced significant movement difficulties after a serious accident. Through imagery, she fully regained her ability to move. Her work is considered foundational by many modern dance schools.[5]

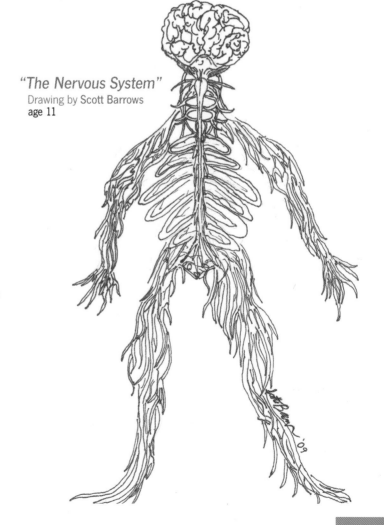

"The Nervous System"
Drawing by Scott Barrows
age 11

[5] Franklin, E. DYNAMIC ALIGNMENT THROUGH IMAGERY

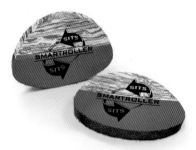

SMARTROLLER® SITS

Use the SITS as kinesthetic learning tools for posture, balance and comfort. These durable pads provide immediate feedback to help distribute your weight onto your sits bones for an optimal sitting experience. A great companion for activities such as yoga and meditation. Set of two. Non-returnable.

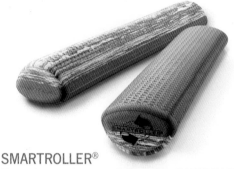

SMARTROLLER®

The revolutionary "two-in-one" shape of the SMARTROLLER makes it one of the most versatile foam rollers available. The rounder side increases roller movement, while the flatter side decreases movement. Made of closed-cell, cross-linked molded foam technology. 4" oblong x 36" long.

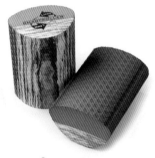

SMARTROLLER® LINKS

Create stable or unstable "links" to address more movement choices during your workout. The LINKS provide a dynamic surface to differentiate and fine-tune body segments. They also make excellent props for Pilates and yoga. 4" oblong x 8 ½" long. Non-returnable.

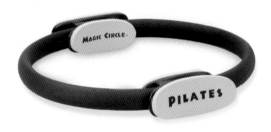

PILATES MAGIC CIRCLE

This soft rubber ring, designed by Joseph Pilates, provides resistance for improving muscle tone and endurance.

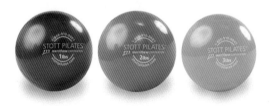

STOTT PILATES® TONING BALLS

These handheld weighted balls from STOTT PILATES are perfect for increasing the challenge level of almost any mat workout. Available in 1-lb., 2-lb. and 3-lb. increments.

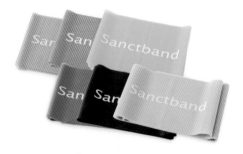

SANCTBAND® PRE-CUT BAND

Add the dynamic resistance of SANCTBAND to your workout. SANCTBAND's new very low powder, reduced protein formula exercise band reduces skin irritation and discomfort caused by powder and protein in natural latex. Available in various pre-cut lengths and rolls.

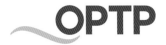